Crow's Feet:
Life As We Age

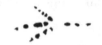

Stories that inspire joy and defy
stereotypes about the last decades of life.

Edited by Nancy Peckenham

Crow's Feet: Life As We Age

Library of Congress Cataloging-in-Publication Data is available.

Print book ISBN 978-1-7352686-0-6

Ebook ISBN 978-1-7352686-1-3

First published October 2020.

Cover photo by Cristian Newman on Unsplash

Part One photo by Nancy Peckenham

Part Two photo by Anthony Metcalfe on Unsplash

Part Three photo by Michelle Cassar on Unsplash

Part Four photo by Markus Spiske on Unsplash

Part Five photo by Nick Karvounis on Unsplash

Part Six photo by Elly Fairytale on Pexels

Cover design by Nancy Peckenham

Typesetting by Fundamental Capabilities Inc.

4/CROW'S FEET

Dedicated to my mother,

Catherine Reilly Peckenham,

whose joy for living in her 100s inspired me

to start *Crow's Feet.*

6/CROW'S FEET

Contents

INTRODUCTION   **11**

PART ONE: Reclaiming What it Means to Age   **15**

The Best Parts   *16*
By Ann Litts

Let's Kick Out the Old Aging Paradigm   *19*
By Beth Bruno

Old Guy Proclamation: Listen Up Whippersnappers!   *22*
By Mark Starlin

The Ageism Problem in Health Care   *23*
By Brittany Denis, DPT

What Does "Looking My Age" Mean?   *29*
By Marie A. Bailey

Why, at Almost 70, I am Redefining Beauty   *32*
By Julia E. Hubbel

PART TWO: Don't Call Me Dear   **37**

Talk to Me When I'm Old   *38*
By Nancy Peckenham

How Not to Talk to A Senior   *39*
By JF Gross

Invisible   *42*
By Dennett

Redundant   46
   By Anne Saddler

What Not to Say to Someone Over 60   50
   By Lili Rodriguez

PART THREE: No Permission Needed   **53**

The Freedom of 50   54
   By Lisa Wathen

Tattoos, Motorcycles and Purple Hair   58
   By Ann Litts

The Freedom of Posing Nude   61
   By Diane Overcash

When I Go Down, It'll Be With a Smile on My Face   65
   By Shea McNaughton

Like a Fine Wine We Get Better with Age   72
   By Michelle Monet

70s – Time to Slow Down?   75
   By DB McNicol

Unlock Your Bias – Old and Grey but We Still Rock   77
   By Caroline de Braganza

PART FOUR: Transitions   **81**

Find Your Superpowers After 50   82
   By Ingrid L. Williams

Five Tips for a Happy Midlife Career Exit   87
   By Kathleen Cardwell

Retirement 92
By Greg Hopkins

How to Age Well and Have Your Best Later Life 95
By Zoe Berry

And the Years Have Flown Away Like the Leaves on a Mid-October Day 100
By Julia E. Hubbel

PART FIVE: An Ounce of Wisdom 105

What Matters 106
By Dennett

Resting in "Being" After a Lifetime of "Doing" 107
By Beth Bruno

How Terribly Not Strange To Be (Almost) Seventy 111
By Paul Hossfield

I Have Lived 80 Years But Have I Learned Anything? 114
By Warren Turner

New Love After Loss – A Valentine of Hope 117
By Katharine Esty, PhD

Life at 102 120
By Nancy Peckenham

PART SIX: Turn Aging On Its Head 123

How Do I Get More Comfortable With That Face in the Mirror? 124
By Mary Dalton Selby

Your Attitudes About Aging Can Predict Your Future   126
    By Brittany Denis, DPT

Looking at Old in a New Way   129
    By Maggie Fry

What Does "Older" Feel Like?   133
    By Nalini MacNab

The Person I Used to Be Came for a Visit   135
    By Anna I. Smith

Why We Should Resist Any Urge to Join the Aging Tribe   139
    By Zoe Berry

Fun with Boomer Barbie   143
    By Roz Warren

AUTHOR BIOGRAPHIES   147

ACKNOWLEDGMENTS   155

INTRODUCTION

It's going to happen to all of us one day, if we're lucky enough to live that long. We will look in the mirror and it will hit us that we have aged. It's a fact of a nature — and one that we can embrace or fear.

Fear of aging comes from a culture that devalues older folks and depicts them as feeble and unproductive. Embracing aging erases these negative stereotypes and allows people to savor the joy and new-found wisdom that comes with each advancing year.

In this collection of essays and poems you will find the voices of women and men who are exploring their own attitudes about aging, shedding outdated images and redefining how we experience life in our final decades. The pieces have been written by people who are delighted with the freedoms they have discovered in their fifties and sixties even as they confront ageist attitudes.

The roots of ageism go deep. Half-a-century ago, men could expect to die in their sixties and women would follow in their early seventies. In popular culture, only the young were endowed with glamour, happiness and adventure, while those older than 60 were thought to be in a slow and steady decline. After people retired from the workplace, they were considered irrelevant.

Today, our understanding of aging has changed. Advances in medical care, along with a parallel movement that emphasizes healthy eating and exercise, have brought new vigor to life in our sixties, seventies and eighties. People feel better, have more energy, and are more active. Each day, each year that older people prosper, we defy the ageist stereotypes of inevitable mental and physical decline.

The stories in this volume show how these changes are occurring. They are written by people from around the world who want to share their excitement in life as they age. They represent a small portion of the 100 writers who are part of *Crow's Feet: Life As We Age,* a publication on *Medium.com,* where the essays and poems first appeared.

At *Crow's Feet,* our mission is to turn aging on its head. We are doing it by shattering negative stereotypes and replacing them with the strength and wisdom that grows with the years. The challenge of deconstructing aging isn't easy. It permeates so many parts of life. But we are raising our voices to be part of the conversation and we will be heard.

The writers in this edition of *Crow's Feet* speak from the frontlines because they write from the heart about their personal experiences with being older, with discovering that their daily lives are filled with both adventures and with a wisdom that allows them to savor life. Their personal stories reveal the lie about aging and prove it to be a fact of life to be embraced, not feared.

In these pages you will find anger and disappointment but also laughter and joy. You will discover truth in the words of Frank Lloyd Wright, who wrote:

"The longer I live the more beautiful life becomes."

14/CROW'S FEET

PART ONE: Reclaiming What it Means to Age

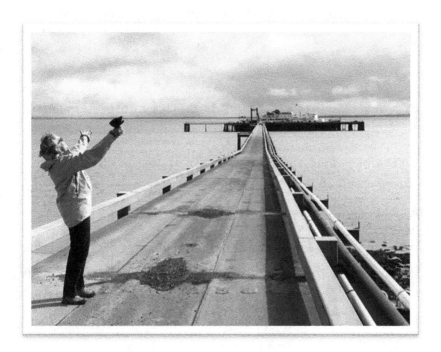

The Best Parts

By Ann Litts

"Growing old is mandatory. Growing up is optional."

Carroll Bryant

Our society likes to focus on youth. This is not breaking news. We bought into the hype all throughout our lifetime.

And now — here we are attempting to undo all the damage it caused to our attitudes on aging.

Because simply stated — this life is not our parent's life.

We are not aging in the same manner as our parents did — in the era prior to the discovery of antibiotics, CT scans, and chemotherapy.

To many of us, aging equals freedom — a fresh start — a new chapter of Life opening up.

The Best Parts of Life.

We are walking away from the day-to-day responsibilities of the 9–5. I can see it — feel it — when I'm around my friends who are retired. The stress of being chained to the profession they choose over twenty years ago is completely gone. We are not the same people we were when we started that career. We long to land in a place where the person we have grown into can flourish, breathe, be let loose. Someplace we *fit.*

We have raised our kids and have morphed into doting grandparents. My daughters still can't figure out how I went from their mother to Nana — the personality change is that significant. We are free to love The Magical Creatures without limits. We know how the story ends — they don't become serial killers if we make a misstep or two along the way. We look at their parents and know someone else is doing the heavy lifting. All we have to provide is Love.

We are downsizing — freeing ourselves of all the shit the kids left behind, moving to warm places, traveling with a lighter load. So many of us are purging. Walking away from all which is not serving us. The collective memorabilia of our lifetimes. Things — relationships — careers. All. The. Things we no longer need/want/use. We are letting go of what needs to go. We are making space for what needs to come. We are finding freedom in simplicity and that less really is more.

We are healthy, vibrant and, yes, still having sex with a partner. Contrary to what the media will have you believe we don't all belong in nursing homes as soon as we hit some magic to-be-determined number. We enjoy all the things we enjoyed doing yesterday — even folks like me who have chronic illnesses.

Aging is not a diagnosis.

Living life right up to the last breath is an attitude. We don't have to buy what the media has been selling us for the last fifty years.

We can politely decline to participate in the gloom and doom which marks "the end of youth" and instead celebrate each and every day, week, month, year we live.

Aging is not the end of life. In fact, for many of us it's just the beginning and holds The Best Parts.

Let's Kick Out the Old Aging Paradigm
It's time to create a new narrative

By Beth Bruno

Do you remember the angst of being a teenager? Every day you looked in the mirror and saw something that looked nothing like the models in those glamour magazines. Between the acne, the braces on your teeth, the awkward body and that hair that refused to cooperate, there was plenty to dislike when you looked in the mirror.

Fast forward to today when you are in your forties, fifties, sixties and beyond. Have you reverted to those same talking points when you look in the mirror? Now you see wrinkles, saggy skin, age spots and hair that refuses to cooperate as it grays and thins. Your teeth aren't as white as they used to be, and *that neck!*

If we continue to parrot the dialogue of the advertisers and the voices in our head, we will find we have a lot to criticize and decry as we age. We have been indoctrinated by a youth-centric society that teaches us from the cradle that the only time in our life we will have any worth is when we are dewy-fresh.

We all know that's not true, but it is hard to overcome the narrative that has been playing over and over our entire lives. We have bought the story and now, as we look at our aging selves in the mirror, we are looking with eyes that can't see our beauty. We see a face and a body that don't measure up, just like we did when we were awkward teenagers.

Yet how many of us would really like to go back to an earlier time in our lives? I know I wouldn't. At 57, this is truly the best time in my life. I know a lot of other women who feel the same way. So how can we begin to reconcile ourselves to the aging face in the mirror and make it a *part* of the story instead of something that we have to be ashamed of, or fix?

While our society still has a long way to go to change its attitude about aging, it's our own attitude toward our very personal aging that has to change the most. If we aren't careful, we will find ourselves sending rude little messages to ourselves about how shameful it is to look like an "old lady." When we get tangled up in the angst that can be created from these messages, we rob ourselves of the joy of these years.

I think we have all had an oh-no! moment when we looked at ourselves and for the first time thought "You look old." If you are like me, after this moment you spend a lot of time obsessing about how you can fix what you see in the mirror in order to go back to looking like you once did. You feel yourself sliding away and this old woman in the mirror taking your place. It can be very disconcerting.

Instead of focusing on the many positives of being an older, wiser and more experienced woman, we are stuck in the mindset of aging as something to fight, something to resist, something to be ashamed of. This wastes a lot of the energy we could be using to go out and make this the best part of our life. This is where facing reality can set us free. As we learn to accept that youth = beauty is an outdated equation, we can begin to formulate a new one.

I finally decided to go with what was happening and learn to embrace it. I decided to let my hair go gray. I accepted that my neck is never going to look like it once did. I am learning to be okay with my eyelids being a little softer and droopier. I am practicing sending myself love every time I stand in front of the mirror or look down at spotted and wrinkled hands. I have worked hard to become this me, and if this is the body that goes along with her, then it deserves my love and respect.

We are lucky that we live in a time when attitudes toward aging are changing and we have so many outstanding role models for aging well. Just a quick Google search will net many stories of older women doing amazing things and sucking all the juice out of their lives, regardless of wrinkles and gray hair. And I know that my grandmother and great-grandmother would be astounded at what women in their fifties and beyond look like today and all the things they are doing with their lives.

We need to create a new model for aging that celebrates the accomplishments of a long life, the many gifts and abilities we still have to share with the world and the ways we have changed and evolved as we have grown older. We need to stop trying to erase the signs of aging and start embracing the amazing women we have become and are continuing to become. It is our turn to define what beauty means.

Look at yourself in the mirror and see what a bad ass you are. Now that's beautiful.

Old Guy Proclamation: Listen Up Whippersnappers!

By Mark Starlin

I wear my graying hair as a badge of honor for time served on this rock
My scars as souvenirs of a life abundantly lived
I am a geezer but not an Ebenezer [Scrooge]
And I am not done yet.

The Ageism Problem in Health Care
And why it impacts all of us

By Brittany Denis, DPT

"It was then that I saw what had been right in front of me my entire career: that the experiences of older people in our health care system are indicative of how current medical care is broken for all of us."

Louise Aronson, Elderhood: Redefining Aging, Transforming Medicine, Reimagining Life

The longer I work in healthcare, the more I encounter blatant ageism throughout the system. I've had patients who have been told that they can't get stronger because of their age, that they will live in pain forever due to their arthritis, and that they shouldn't stay active because they might fall. These are all examples of false statements spread by authority figures that cause harm.

And taking it a step further, older adults are discriminated against if they use an assistive device to walk, even by their medical providers. It's automatically assumed all older adults are hard of hearing, causing people to shout at them. They get called "cute" or are addressed by demeaning names such as "honey" or "sweetie." Again, all examples of ageist stereotypes being propagated by the very people who should know better.

This is a reflection of an issue that's larger than healthcare. Much of the ageism we encounter within the medical community stems from the ageism that runs rampant throughout society.

The Shortage of Providers for Older Adults

Our first indication of the ageism issue in healthcare is how few providers want to specialize in medicine for older adults. And that translates into poor quality of care for this age group. Older adults are a specialty population in medicine, but not for the reasons most people think.

As Louise Aronson, a gerontologist, highlights in her book *Elderhood*, older adults make up 16% of the population but over 40% of hospitalized adults. Patients over the age of 65 are the group most likely to be harmed by medical care.

According to the American Geriatric Society, there are almost 3,600 full-time practicing geriatricians. But for adequate care for the 14 million older adults living today, we need at least 20,000 practicing geriatricians. The gap between availability and demand is wide, despite geriatricians reporting the highest job satisfaction among physicians.

In the few years I worked as a physical therapist in a skilled nursing facility, I saw the implications of this day in and day out. The lack of knowledge among healthcare providers about how to properly treat older adults leads to two major issues.

Older Adults Are Being Over-Treated And Under-Treated At The Same Time.

As medical providers, we are trained to identify problems and treat them, which is difficult for problems that don't have obvious solutions. Medications and surgical interventions are obvious; these are solutions with more guidelines and indications. But this translates into over-medicating older adults.

The solutions that are often most essential and translate into the best outcomes, like access to a community, adequate transportation, physical mobility, and healthy meals are issues that aren't so easily solved — so they go overlooked. Most of the solutions for these issues are not even offered because of the difficulty in implementing them and the lack of reimbursement for such services. And this is when the mistreatment of older adults harms all of us. We limit access to the most impactful services, despite their relatively low cost compared to expensive medical treatments. We've deemed these issues as too complicated to solve because they are not as simple as prescribing medication.

The Promotion of Aging Myths Within Healthcare

The second indication of ageism throughout healthcare is the rampant promotion of aging stereotypes from healthcare providers treating older adults.

At the start of this article, I mentioned examples of false statements spread by healthcare providers to their patients. It's harmful and untrue to tell someone their strength can't improve because they are 80 years old. The reality is that we start to see strength decline as early as age 30 or 40. Improving strength is a matter of practice and repetition, which can happen at any age.

There isn't anything about aging that limits us from improving, but we've been instilled with the belief that this isn't true. The truth is that you can build muscle, learn new skills, and continue to grow well into your later years.

Healthcare providers tend to miscalculate risk vs. benefit, leading them to tell their older adult patients to limit situations in which they "might fall." And most of the time this advice is recommended without performing a physical fall screening to identify an at-risk patient before offering advice.

While it's true that falls do become more common as we age, it has more to do with behavior change that comes along with aging. And that behavior change is often caused by ageist beliefs. We limit our activity a little every year because of some misguided belief that we are "too old to…"

The truth is that frailty isn't inevitable. You may develop arthritis as you age, but it doesn't mean you have to live a life of limited mobility and pain. You might fall, but we all fall at some point. The benefits of staying active outweigh the risk of falling. Your physical health can continue to improve with age so long as you continue to practice. And this is what we *should* be hearing from our healthcare providers.

What You Can Do

"Unlike other prejudices such as racism and sexism… ageism is unique in targeting our future selves."

Ashton Applewhite

So, where does this leave us? Changes within healthcare are needed at the levels of systems and policy, but change is also dependent on changing individual beliefs. It's up to all of us to start to change the culture of ageism, not just in healthcare but in all settings.

Here's where to start:

Educate Yourself on Ageism

It's hard to identify ageism if we don't understand what is true of aging and what are aging myths. Learn more about changes that come with aging and how aging is viewed in our society.

Reading more about aging and ageism is a good start. I recommend *Elderhood: Redefining Aging, Transforming Medicine, and Reimagining Life* by Louise Aronson; *This Chair Rocks: A Manifesto Against Ageism* by Ashton Applewhite; and *Dynamic Aging* by Katy Bowman to challenge your perception of aging.

Identify Your Own Aging Bias

Whether or not we want to admit it, we all live with some kind of aging bias. And it's difficult to shed these misguided beliefs when we live in a society that promotes "anti-aging."

Start to observe your own thoughts on aging and see if they are in alignment with the reality of aging. Are they mostly positive or negative thoughts? We can't start to resolve the systemic issues of ageism until we learn to recognize our own ageist beliefs.

Create Learning Moments with Others

We can't solve a problem we aren't talking about. It's important to move the conversation beyond researching, learning, and identifying our own internal beliefs.

It can be difficult, but calmly correct others who are spreading misinformation on aging or ageist beliefs. Most people aren't aware they are causing harm. Approach these situations carefully and try to help others learn through discussion.

Solving the broader issues of ageism starts at the individual level. Both the young and the old need to be on board because ageism impacts us all. More voices are needed in this space to facilitate change. Learn what you can, identify your own ageist beliefs, and be an advocate for yourself within the healthcare system.

What Does "Looking My Age" Mean?
And tell me why I should care

By Marie A. Bailey

Seriously, just what do people mean when they use the phrase "look your age?" For context, I'm sixty-two years old, and I still don't understand what looking my age is supposed to look like.

As a kid, I heard the women in my family criticize other women for keeping their hair long and dark past a certain age. Not looking their age was considered scandalous. I never knew where that line was drawn, but I know that's one reason why I chafe at the thought of "looking my age." I just don't know what it means but it sounds prescriptive.

Rebel that I am, I look however I want to. If that means dressing in long black skirts and sensible shoes, my hair short and gray, sure, why not, if it's what suits me at the moment? But it could also mean dressing in yoga tights, a colorful tunic, and Birkenstock sandals, my hair a braided peacock feather.

But that isn't quite it, is it? It's not how I choose to dress or how I style my hair. Looking my age at this time of my life probably means I have wrinkles, crow's feet, laugh lines. My skin is less elastic and sags where I least want it to sag. Little hard white bumps appear and disappear on my skin. I developed rosacea in my late fifties, a particularly cruel diagnosis after battling pimples and blackheads most of my young adult life.

As women, we get mixed messages about how we should look. The messages come both from the media and each other. On one hand, we're prompted to indulge our desire for youthful appearance and buy cosmetics or treatments that promise ageless beauty. On the other, we're encouraged to wear our wrinkles, our dull and sagging skin, like some kind of badge. Go ahead and use Botox if it makes you feel better, but you know you earned those wrinkles.

Ashton Applewhite, author of the *This Chair Rocks: A Manifesto Against Ageism,* captures this tension in an interview with *The Sydney Morning Herald*:

"If you've got to do it, you've got to do it, but in the broader sense, as long as we do these things, we reinforce age shame; the idea that these natural transitions are shameful; the idea that our bodies are betraying us simply because they are changing; the idea that wrinkles are ugly."

Further compounding the "damned if you do, damned if you don't" mixed message about beauty and aging, we have women in their forties being lauded for "looking their age."

I've got nothing against women in their forties. That was a good decade for me. I have very fond memories of my forties. No, it's just that our society is so ageist that even women who are considered middle-aged are being written about as if they were much older.

However, while I enjoyed my forties and fifties, I do remember that my thirties were a time of anxiety, self-doubt, and fear. The fear that loomed the most was the fear of growing old.

Young women are not being encouraged to embrace aging, to see getting older as on par with getting stronger and more self-confident, to see each decade of life as an unfolding of new opportunities, hopes, and dreams.

No, we can't be free to *just* grow older, to *just* try and be healthy and enjoy the freedom that older age can bring. No, our society demands that older women have to be desirable as well. By all means, become a marathon runner when you're in your seventies. Take up mountain climbing in your eighties. Start a new business in your nineties. Look your age while you're at it, but also look desirable.

I have a feeling this wrinkle in our society's ageist view of aging won't be ironed out in what remains of my lifetime. So, don't mind me if I settle for how I feel about myself and ignore how I look to others. I'm just too old to be bothered.

Why, at Almost 70, I am Redefining Beauty

On letting go of the past and embracing what's coming

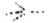

By Julia E. Hubbel

What do you and I do, particularly as women, as the Goddess begins to work Her magic on our faces, our bodies and our beings as we age?

What do you and I do, as women, when we are forced to face the inevitability of our Becoming? As we must let go of what defined us as girls, as mothers, as creatures of desire?

What happens?

I can't speak for anyone else. I've never been a great beauty. Never was. Once in my long life, when I was in my early thirties, I got that kind of attention. I'd starved myself stick thin. I had on a white silk dress with red dots, which was being played around my body by the breeze whipping around the buildings in Washington, DC. I got a wolf whistle.

I'M NOT THAT GIRL ANYMORE.

Never will be again.

Some would say that I was in my prime back then.

I wouldn't. Not with the sexual assaults, the rapes, the eating disorders, the terrible psychic pain. Prime? Please. Just...*please*.

My prime is just beginning.

Perhaps what is most important about barking at 70, just a few years away, is that the girl who still lives inside me, for she does, who used to cry out for that kind of acknowledgement, has finally just sat down.

She had her time in the sun.

ANOTHER, DEEPER PART OF ME IS JUST BEGINNING TO STAND UP.

You and I, especially at this age, are the sum of all the women* we have been, the personalities and roles we have inhabited, the personas and masks we wore. We are, at this age, able to dip a brush into any of the pots of our previous lives and, from them, begin to draw who we can become. This is how the Goddess paints us.

She can do little if we are forever staring into the vessel that contained us in our youth, our gazes full of woe, loss, and longing, and false memories of a "better time." How quickly we forget our youthful angst, our terror about aging, the night sweats about the wrinkles. The fear that we'd lose our value as we aged.

We lose our value when we mourn our youth and fail to step into the promise of our legacy.

The Goddess offers a partnership.

My job is to keep the body, mind and spirit strong and limber.

And to stay open.

The Goddess would like to deliver gifts. Among them: light, in the heart, in the soul, and a lighter burden as we shed what no longer matters.

The Goddess' greatest gift: *humor.* For as we do indeed face that good night, the gentility and grace that come with our ability to laugh is our greatest guarantee that you and I will live well, for however long we have left.

As we age into ourselves, our promise, it's available to let go of all the attachments and identifications with our bodies, the currency of youth or beauty or both. Some of us age very well and continue to be stunning well into our eighties and beyond. Externally, at least.

For my part, whether or not I continue to sport physical beauty is nowhere near as important as whether I have the courage to let life carve itself into my face.

Whether I can continue to rise, then stand, then revel in what my final years offer me. The chance to know freedom. The potential to grow wisdom. To continue to dip into those paint pots and create the masterpiece that is whatever legacy I might leave.

I have no idea what that might be. I do know, and strongly believe, that once we pass sixty, the last decades of our lives might best be spent not only in gratitude for making it this far, but in giving back from the living bible of our own experiences.

Those parts of me that no longer serve, *I have sat them down*.

For I must, or else be slave to the demands of those lesser parts of me that clamor for my attention, at a time when I have limited time and attention to give.

As women, as Women of Age, the opportunity is to blaze our own trail through the aging process. Nobody can possibly do what you can do in the world. You and I have gifts. Those gifts, left unexpressed, rob the larger world of your footprints. For many of us, the path ahead is long and wide and inviting.

The question is whether we will spend the years that the Goddess is weaving silver into our hair aching for youth and beauty or a long-lost waistline, identifying with what is no longer. And in some cases, never was.

Or, you and I can be painted by a loving Goddess, in all the colors of our exquisite potential, unleashed when we release our youth.

How will the world feel your footprints?

This is of course as true for men as for women, but I'm talking to the ladies at the moment.

PART TWO: Don't Call Me Dear

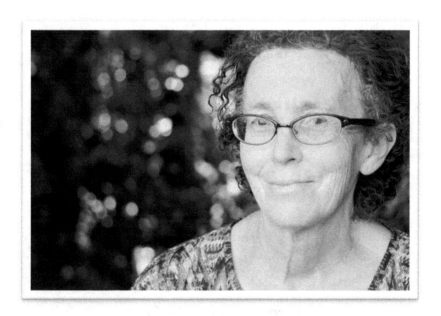

Talk to Me When I'm Old

By Nancy Peckenham

Talk to me like I'm not there,
And I will disappear.

Talk about me, in front of me, a piece of furniture,
And I will withdraw, resentful.

The glazed look in my eyes will be a shield
Against your stupidity.

I'm not deaf and I sure am not dumb.
I just can't remember what I ate for breakfast.

Tell me a story and I will feel
The same passions you do.
My feelings have not evaporated
with my short-term memory.

I am living. I am alive.
Talk to me.

How Not to Talk to A Senior

By JF Gross

I just turned 70 and, apparently, if I died now it wouldn't be too soon. That's not meant as a putative friend might say, "*She* didn't die a moment too soon," but as the seemingly universal opinion that dying as early as mid-sixty is not a life short-changed. That's old age and that's what old people do. They die, they watch TV, they shuffle around the block in the morning dragging their old dogs. And if you run into them on their walk, remember: the only two topics of conversation are the weather and their little rat terrier.

I realized I was considered old when people — doctors, neighbors, cashiers, librarians — started calling me "dear." And along with the "dear" came greatly scaled-down conversations.

It was the same thing every day and multiple times a day: "Think we'll get more rain?" and "How old is your dog?" The forecast question was usually followed by the stale adage, "If you don't like the weather, wait a minute." Not because they'd forgotten they said it just the day before but because they thought *I* would forget.

I remember once reading a short story about a man so bored by his luncheon companion that he fell asleep face first in his soup. You can take only so much.

When and why did this start? Don't these people realize I'm of the Woodstock Generation? Though I didn't make it to the festival because my friends and I spent all our money — $15 — on the one in Atlantic City two weeks before. And drugs. But we still saw Janis Joplin, Jefferson Airplane and the Mothers of Invention. Care to talk about Janis? That was the heyday of grass and hash, and acid safe enough to drop, which we did every Friday, as soon as our campus-cafeteria jobs ended so we wouldn't waste a minute of our weekend. It's a wonder I made the Dean's List. Or earned a degree. And moved to Boulder before it was *Boulder*, before the Pearl Street Mall.

Or we could talk about the Vietnam War protests I attended on the University of Colorado campus, or encircling Rocky Flats, or washing clothes alongside Allen Ginsberg at the laundromat near my house. My sister and I heard Gloria Steinem speak at CSU not long after she launched *Ms.* magazine and saw Angela Davis at Loretto Heights College after her release from prison. We were the only Caucasians in the audience and had our purses confiscated but then cordially returned when (we guessed) no weapons were uncovered.

Half of the '70s and part of the '80s I spent at a left-wing daily where the staff brought their dogs to work and my toddler slept in the office during the long overnight shifts. We were midway into pasting up the paper one night when an editor broke the news that John Lennon had just been shot. I tore apart the front page and rebuilt it with the new lead as we took Little Feat off the shop stereo and played "Imagine" into the morning. I was at *The Denver Post* the day Columbine happened and it stayed on the front page for months, the beginning of mass-shooting stories.

After a large-scale downsizing at the *Post* I had to start over in my fifties, leaving behind a three-decade-long career.

But the old are resilient. Take my little terrier. We've trekked a thousand trails together and still hike every afternoon. She was fast enough once to catch a chipmunk though I always tried to distract her. But she's snagged only five in 15 years so it wasn't exactly genocide. On one hike *she* was the prey, when she wandered off-trail and a trio of coyotes attacked. They fled when I crashed through the trees louder than a mother bear, but her wounds soaked us both as I raced uphill to the car, imagining a heart attack and a murder-suicide headline.

We survived, her stitches healed, and she doesn't think twice about chasing rabbits, though she does weigh the effort for squirrels. She's learned they'll just scale the nearest tree. But that's not infirm, that's pragmatic. With age comes wisdom.

So the next time you're tempted to talk about the weather — wait a minute. Then, don't.

Invisible
Aging in the workplace

By Dennett

(Inspired by a co-worker who feels marginalized

because of her age.)

30 years —
I've done this for 30 years,
It's a profession, not a job —
My profession.
I communicate, coordinate, correlate, translate, and delegate,
Transforming paper mountains into legal transactions —

I can make a house your home, a spouse your ex,
Help you prepare for a new life or death,
Turn a passion into a business,
Turn a liability into an asset.

I contact, contract, transact and redact,
Sometimes a glorified secretary,
Sometimes a paralegal,

Always a professional.

My work is exemplary,
My ethics impeccable,
Always efficient,
Always busy,
Always here.

I'm 56 —
Not sickly,
Not demented,
Not confused.

My memory sharp,
My skills perfected,
My knowledge legendary.

I do more than
Young ones who do less
And want more.

I care more than
Young ones who
Couldn't care less.

I am quicker, wiser, smarter
And don't trade on good looks
And fast promises.

So, why do you
Negate
Isolate
Discriminate
Intimidate
Displace
Replace
Me?

As though I am no one,
As though I gave nothing —
I gave all,
I am still giving all.

But I've been replaced
Without quitting or
Firing or retiring.
My experience displaced
By youth and inexperience.

Yet, here I stay,
Working,
Unappreciated
Unrewarded

Unnoticed.

30 years and
I've become invisible.

Redundant

A woman in her fifties laments her loss of status.

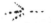

By Anne Saddler

I stare through the rain-streaked window.
Everything is grey.
The low cloud dampens my mood, slows my mind.
I stay in bed.
Warm tea in my mug, warm dog nestled between my knees.
Nothing to get up for.

My witch-mother prophesied:

When a woman hits fifty, an invisible mantle descends from the
ether to veil her...obscure her. Once cloaked, her light grows
dim, her presence dwindles, she begins to fade into the
background. Her presence diminished, she sinks slowly into
obscurity. Believe me, she said. You'll see, she said. Mark my
words.

I watch the Gulls.
They swirl, and twirl, in the stilled, salted air.
Strangely silent, they wait for the cloud to lift.

They come each week; they know it's Tuesday.
Below the fog, dustbins filled with promise
Line the streets like rows of blackened teeth.
There's easy pickings to be had from rotting mouths.
If I were a gull, I'd get in there first, tear at the bags,
Make my chances,
Pick out the best.
I wouldn't share.
Playing nice doesn't get you anywhere.

My mother warned me. I didn't listen.
It'll be different for me, I thought.
I'm strong, work hard. I'm respected, admired.
I toe the line, give my best, they know my worth.
I'll shrug the cloak from my capable shoulders.
I'll brush the suffocating heaviness of 50 off, like dandruff.
These are my days, not yours...
Things have changed, Mother.
The fifth decade, the cursed benefactress of maturity;
Ambition blinded by age.
Its eyes put out by crow's feet, grey hairs, hot-flushes-in-
important-meetings,
And the need to be in bed by 22:30.
Capability? No longer recognized.
Knowledge? Now largely ignored.
Opinions? Un-sought, or worse, unwelcome.
Aspirations? Sidelined for new projects.
Ambition? Overlooked for new jobs — no promotion.

"Hello? Hello? Can nobody see me?"

Nature sticks the knife in deeper...and twists.
The comfy nest flown without a backward glance.
Looks compromised by bleeding lipstick,
Flats instead of heels,
Used-up hormones. Cobweb brain.
The dis-in-ter-est-ed partner.

White and cream houses dot the far side of the valley.
They hover on a marshmallow of pinky-grey sea mist,
Empty shells with no souls.
Their occupants left for work an hour ago.
A busy commute, a full diary.
Compliant automatons on their daily grind.
I wonder if, like me, someone across the valley is lying in bed,
Abandoned, with warm tea, and a dog, and no future.

I think about the day ahead — there's no reason to stir.
I inherited my mother's cloak and disappeared along with my
successes.
I've nothing to do, no-one to see.
No Inbox now I'm out.
Purposeless, worthless, pointless, redundant,
I'm useless; of-no-use.

May as well stay here then...in bed,
With warm tea in my mug, and warm dog nestled between my
knees.
I stare through the rain-streaked window,
And everything is grey.

What Not to Say to Someone Over 60

Calling someone "young lady" who is 30 years your senior isn't cute

By Lili Rodriguez

If you're over the age of 60, and especially if you're female, this has probably happened to you. You're sitting at a table in a restaurant, or you're approached by a salesperson in a store, and your 20-something waiter or salesperson says, "What can I get for you, young lady?" Or "there you go, young lady" while placing your order on the table.

Young lady? WTF?

Apparently, I've gotten old enough that I'm somehow "cute" to young people who see me as a doddering old relic from the Mesozoic era. (That's when dinosaurs roamed the earth, for those who have a gaping hole in their education about earth's history).

They think it's cute to call me "young lady," which, when said to someone over 60 by someone under 30, actually means "You're an incredibly old lady. How amazing that a person as old as you still goes out to dinner or tries to buy things in a store." Or maybe "you remind me of my darling old granny who can't be trusted to leave the house alone."

I would assume this happens to men as well, but I would bet they have to be significantly older (e.g., over 70 or 80) to get a "What can I get for you, young man?"

Referring to someone 30 years your senior as "young lady" or "young man" is, in reality, a way to signify that they no longer really count. They're no longer a vital, vibrant, attractive, intelligent person with a full life and a future ahead of them. They're over the hill, headed for the dustbin. Or, for men, that they're no longer virile. They've become nothing but an "old man."

Would you call an obviously overweight person "skinny"? As in "hey skinny — how can I help you?".

My entire career is based on my ability to understand why people do what they do. As a consumer researcher and cultural anthropologist, understanding people is what I do for a living. But I can't for the life of me understand what goes through the mind of a person who calls me "young lady," especially in the service industry where, presumably, they expect they might get a tip if they do a good job.

I guess they think I'll be flattered, or amused. But would anyone seriously think a woman in her sixties would be flattered by a person in their twenties calling them "young lady"? On any level you think about it, calling me "young lady" is right on the edge of outright sarcasm.

Here's a tip from someone on the far side of 60 direct to those Millennials who think calling me "young lady" is cute. It's not cute. Not even a bit cute. It's condescending and offensive, and if I thought I could get away with it I'd slap your face or wash your mouth out with soap for saying it.

PART THREE: No Permission Needed

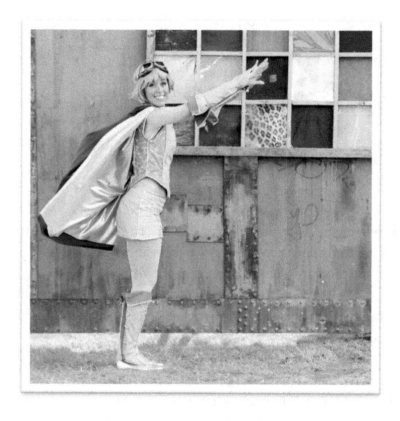

The Freedom of 50

What gifts does the fifth decade of life bring?

By Lisa Wathen

"It's amazing what passing the half-century mark does to free one to be eccentric."

Madeleine L'Engle, A Circle of Quiet

I've been waiting to lay claim to midlife eccentricity since I first read these words as a 14-year-old girl. It sounded like heaven: turn 50, and all the pressures and tethers and expectations of how to be a woman will be cut loose, and you're free to be weird, your quirks and peculiarities — which used to mark you as a misfit or someone who *could* be attractive if she'd just put in a little effort — become assets.

Maybe they even make you a little fascinating.

I imagined myself literally skipping and running through a sunlit field of flowers, my hair a graying mess, my clothes ill-fitting and mismatched, a glorious smile on my face as I leave behind any hint of caring what other people think of me, eager to pursue my own agenda for the second half of my life.

I really thought it'd be as simple as that: one day I'd lift my head from my pillow and be transformed into a woman who is no longer touched by all the things that weighed me down for the previous five decades. Poof! Welcome to the ball, Cinderella!

However, much has changed in our world since 1972, when Madeleine L'Engle was writing. I think that 50 was older then. There was no expectation that women should present themselves as sexually active, ambitious members of mainstream society as they aged.

Today, women have a much bigger voice in society. We have a considerable and growing presence in government and the work force. The assumption that we will stay home with the children is vanishing. The acknowledgement and valuing of women over 30, their wisdom, productivity, and attractiveness has grown. "Over the Hill" isn't such a thing anymore, as we age.

And so, in this modern context, I revisit Madeleine's observations and wonder if there's any truth in them for me.

My 49th birthday is a few days away, and while that's not 50, it does mark the beginning of my fifth decade of life. Even in this very different landscape of what it means to be a woman, I have waited so long, anticipated with such eager hope, the freedom she wrote about. For weeks now I have been looking for signs of that shivering transformation.

The Reality Of Getting Older.

Well, I'm certainly not cavorting through fields of flowers. I don't feel untethered from responsibility, daily life demands, or meeting the needs of others. I'm definitely not free to do just as I please and let the rest of the world go hang. All of which was, I thought all those years ago, part of the midlife gig for women like Madeleine and me.

To be fair, I don't think Madeleine meant that at all. She had many work and daily life chores and obligations to answer to throughout her long life. Part of what she writes about in *A Circle of Quiet* is her need to find escape from the pressure of it all, even in her late fifties, space and time to regain healthy perspective and nourish her soul with alone time, with nature, with her own thoughts.

But I also think there is a deeper truth to what she meant, one that I could not have understood as a fledgling woman all those years ago.

At The Heart Of It

Three and a half decades later, I have learned something about what truly matters to me and, I think, *that* is what Madeleine meant: knowing what to pare away from the daily serving of to-do's without guilt or second-guessing my choices, without worrying whether I'm right or wrong, because I just know what's *most important.*

For Madeleine it was not caring how she looked as she tramped across the fields to find her quiet place and get away from the *sturm und drang* of family life for a while. It was also giving herself permission to take that piece of time for herself, setting aside any qualms about being an insufficient housewife because she had come to know that it was less important than her sense of balance, her need for quiet and meditation. Probably she'd learned the hard way that doing anything else resulted in misery for everyone.

So, there it is, the midlife grace that blesses us in our fifties: lessons taught by time and life experience. Different for each of us, they bring freedom because they release us from having to learn those particular lessons anymore. We've got it now. We can move on to the next thing.

I have no doubt there are new lessons to be learned. As I think back over the past five decades, there are many things I wish I could tell my younger self— if only I could spare myself some of the sorrow and difficulty! It seems almost a certainty that at some distant, future time I'll think back to me, now, and wish I could do the same for my cusp-of-50-self.

That's all right. I accept that it's axiomatic that we often have to learn things the hard way. I am armed with all the lessons I've mastered so far, I'm free of the old blind spots and ignorance and ready to tackle new territory.

I think I'll go put on a lumpy old hat, my favorite stretched out sweatshirt and those corduroy pants I found at a sidewalk sale in Philadelphia in 2003, and stride out into the rainy winter afternoon, to thump and splash through puddles and breathe in the day, not giving a thought to what the neighbors might think or whether or not I should be inside cooking or cleaning or grading papers.

My five decades have taught me that those *shoulds* don't matter. And so, like Madeleine, I'm going to revel in my freedom.

Tattoos, Motorcycles and Purple Hair

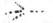

By Ann Litts

I was a quiet child. No, it's true. I got good grades, did all the Right Things. I tried desperately to make friends and fit in.

Right up until the time I didn't.

Somewhere around 50 — I found Her. The person I had been all along. She was here, just waiting for me to grow up. Catch up. Mature. Grow a set.

Become Real.

I found My Real Life in Middle Age. Nearly everything about me has changed in the last 18 years. In *"Juicy Tomatoes: Plain Truths, Dumb Lies, and Sisterly Advice about Life after 50,"* Susan Swartz calls estrogen a domesticating hormone. Once I was free of its influence, Wild came into My Life like a runaway train.

I simply had to be Free. There was no other choice. It was imperative.

I became bolder, braver, fiercer. I got divorced. I got a tattoo. Then two more. I got a motorcycle license. Then a motorcycle. For the last three years, I've had purple hair — because my cousin dared me at a family reunion and my granddaughter told me to go with purple. No one for a minute thought I'd keep it this long. Except perhaps my stylist — who knows me better than my therapist.

I found a voice. My Voice. I started writing. First, in a journal — journals of poison poured out of me. Then at last — on *Medium* where The Universe led me.

I stopped taking responsibility for things that belonged to others. I minded My Own Life — My Own Feelings — My Own Path.

I had found My Edges — fortified My Boundaries — and held them fast.

And in doing so — the most amazing thing happened to me. I ceased to care what anyone thought about me. I didn't care at all if they thought I was smart or pretty or well-dressed or crazy or vulgar or poor or young — well — just pick a thing. You catch my drift.

The Freedom which comes from being in this place is completely exhilarating.

Some days it still will take my breath away. The Complete Joy of it.

I'm turning sixty this year. I have made friends with My Body. Yoga and meditation practices help me balance All. The. Things. I am not without chronic health issues that remind me I am an eternal being having a human experience. One day I will have to say goodbye to My Friend — My body.

But Today — Today — We Live.

Getting older isn't for sissies, as the saying goes. It's for the bold — the brave — the fierce among us. The Real.

"It doesn't happen all at once,' said the Skin Horse. 'You become. It takes a long time. That's why it doesn't happen often to people who break easily, or have sharp edges, or who have to be carefully kept. Generally, by the time you are Real, most of your hair has been loved off, and your eyes drop out and you get loose in the joints and very shabby. But these things don't matter at all, because once you are Real you can't be ugly, except to people who don't understand.'"

Margery Williams Bianco, The Velveteen Rabbit

Namaste.

The Freedom of Posing Nude

The last time was when I was 56 years old.

By Diane Overcash

It's freezing out here. The nipples are crinkling in protest. Never mind trying to hide, little brown buttons. We are in this together.

Angela is already marching down the road ahead of me with her newly acquired early-Christmas-present camera looking for a picturesque spot for me to pose. She and her husband own this bit of acreage, so we don't expect any interruptions. At least there is that.

This is Angela's idea, but it didn't take much to talk me into it. I've known her for years. She is an accomplished painter and a gifted photographer. She is also a little bit crazy. The good kind of crazy.

So here we are in the early morning of late October tromping through the woods. One of us is naked as the day she was born. It is exciting.

Angela had the idea to take pictures of real women, paint them life-size and create a gallery show. She wanted to show what real women look like, with lumps and bumps, Cesarean scars, stretch marks and the lot. I thought it was a brilliant idea. "I'm all in," I told her. I am the fifth one of her subjects for this ambitious undertaking.

She posed me sitting on a large bolder, my legs crossed, and hands draped across my knees, my face turned left gazing into the far-off distance. She said she loved my sweet smile that looked like I was hiding a secret.

Next, I am standing beside a huge oak, one hand outstretched leaning on the tree. I placed the other hand on my hip, one knee bent throwing my hip forward. Isn't this how the Greek goddesses posed? I think it might be.

I don't have a runway model type of body. I am medium height with a large behind and a small waist. The pear shape they call it. My weight fluctuates. Sometimes, I can be described as being plump as a partridge. In this instance, I am more gazelle than partridge.

This is not my first rodeo appearing nude in public. I posed for drawing class when I was in college. I enjoyed it. I thought it was modern and edgy. I was in art school, after all. I didn't see anything wrong with it. I still don't.

I was good at posing. My classmates told me I was one of the best models they had. I could hold a pose for long periods of time. Very important when you are drawing. And I could choose poses that were interesting to draw. I imagined what I would like to see if I were doing the drawing.

Out here in these woods with my friend, I feel a profound sense of freedom. I feel appreciated and beautiful as she walks from side to side to find the best light. Camera pointed at me, I am the focus of her attention.

We walked down a dirt road chatting about art, her eyes scanning the horizon for good light.

"Look up there at the top of that embankment. There's a big rock. Climb up there and sit on that rock. That will be a great shot from down below."

"Up there? Well, OK."

I started the long scramble up the sliding-dirt hill. My arms and legs were spraddled out like a spider climbing a wall. My nether parts were aimed in her direction.

Do you even have to ask? Yes, hell yes, of course, she took the picture. And it is one of my favorites. Back lighting blurred the questionable sections. All you can see is shapes. It's beautiful. I snort with laughter every time I see it. It brings me such joy.

Angela hasn't finished the paintings. In the perfectly unpredictable Angela way, she gets great ideas and seldom finishes them. Maybe she gets them finished as much as she needs to.

It wouldn't be out of character for her to get these paintings finished in the far-distant future.

This makes two times in my life where I put myself out there for all the world to see. Some people wouldn't like it. I was willing to accept that.

At these times I felt fully alive. I felt like the world was balanced and spinning on its axis as it should be.

When I Go Down, It'll Be With a Smile on My Face

Because living in fear is for sissies.

By Shea McNaughton

"And in the end, it's not the years in your life that counts. It's the life in your years."

Edward J. Stieglitz

I ride motorcycle.

To be honest, I ride in the thickly cushioned backseat with side speakers, a cup holder for my pink sparkly monogrammed beverage cup (thanks, Honey), fully wired to the gentleman in the driver's seat.

I'm not a thrill seeker, an adrenaline junkie, or even terribly brave. I am, however, addicted to adventure. And riding motorcycle is a thrill like no other.

I'm this way because I turned 60 years old this year. I've had a decent life. Lots of travel in my younger years and my fair share of heartache. I survived a relationship so toxic and abusive that my cardiologist told me it shortened my life by five years.

But now it's time to face the music – I ain't gettin' any younger.
Until four years ago, I was bulletproof. I could lose weight when I wanted, merely by eating less and speed-walking to China and back on the treadmill every evening while carrying 3-lb. hand weights. My hair was thick and strong. And I slept well at night. I was single and quite happy to be so.

Then I fell into the greasy, toxic slime pit known as a relationship with a covert, malignant narcissist, and it all changed. I gained 30 pounds, my hair fell out, I stopped sleeping and my heart decided to strike up the big brass band at odd times of the day or night. Oh, and my blood pressure skyrocketed too.

So, I dumped his sorry ass.

I was 59 years old. And my relationship bank account was bone dry empty. Again. I was on my own with no one to play with. No one to have my back. No one to watch movies with, go dancing with, or sleep with. No one to eat with, and no one to hold my hand. No one to tell me he loved me.

I was completely and utterly alone. And I f---ing loved it!
Do you know how liberating it is to drag your battered soul out from under the crushing weight of a deadbeat "lover?" Someone who takes and takes and takes but never gives? Someone who almost literally sucks the life out of you?

Survival will do that to you. It'll make you relish each day like it could be your last. Carpe f—ing diem. There's no freedom quite like it.

And that was when I decided that the rest of my life would be devoted to adventure.

I don't mean the kind of adventure that comes from scaling Mt. Everest or running with the bulls at Pamplona. Or even the adventure of traveling solo to a foreign country.

For one thing, stratospheric altitude isn't for the likes of this recovering computer potato. I prefer gentler cows to bulls. And traveling solo just doesn't sound like much fun to me — I want to share the experiences with someone close to me.

No, I'm talking about adventure right in my own back yard, so to speak. Taking road trips by myself. Learning to shoot a better game of pool. Joining a singing group. Getting involved with the local arts council. And enjoying the very act of being single and older, which to many is a terrifying state, but which to me was heaven on earth.

And then I met someone…and he rides motorcycle.

I hadn't "biked" in 10 years, and even then, it was only for a couple of hours here and there, skipping from bar to bar on the back of a city bike. (He drank diet soda. I drank fun stuff.) The kind of bike designed for the driver, but not so much for a passenger. The kind that had a tiny 11"x11" passenger "seat" on the back, kind of like an afterthought.

Compared to how I ride now (and the gentleman with whom I ride), that was a little pastel pony compared to a thoroughbred racehorse.

This is riding on steroids. From Texas to Colorado and back in 2,300 miles of rain, snow, blistering heat and high altitude, on highways and tiny back roads. Now that's riding motorcycle.

You should hear the doom-and-gloomers:
"It's not a question of 'if' but 'when.' "

"My parents had an accident once — they picked glass out of their skin for weeks."

"You should hear my wife's stories from the ER of people in motorcycle accidents."

And my personal favorite… "Oh my gosh, at YOUR age?!?"

Yeah, yeah, I know. Somehow motorcycling is seen as the greatest personal danger of all time. And it's true in a sense — drivers of full-size vehicles often don't see bikes and bikers. We're small and we don't take up visual space like full-size vehicles do, which is why bikers need to be extra vigilant.

The seasoned vets are. They have to watch out for the oncoming driver who wants to "make the light," even after it turned red two seconds ago. They have to watch for the folks who check their blind spots in the mirror but don't turn their heads to make sure. And they'd better watch out for sleepy or otherwise preoccupied truckers who are in a hurry to make deadlines.

Still, there's nothing quite like the thrill of riding at 70 mph in the open air with only two wheels beneath you and nothing overhead. It's the thrilling equivalent of dining al fresco.

Traveling by motorcycle thrusts you headfirst into your road trip.
It's the only way to smell "road perfume," whether it's skunk in the country, roses in the suburbs, fast food grease in the city or the occasional ripe fragrance of roadkill.

Riding to the top of Pike's Peak, a steep sinewy strip of asphalt curling 'round the mountain and marked with constant hairpin turns with nary a guardrail in sight, left my stomach so tangled in knots that only three pieces of Rocky Mountain fudge could unwind it.

Why do I do this? Why not spend my "golden years" in more sedate pursuits?

Screw the "Golden Years."
I do this...

- because my children are grown and on their own.

- because all of my financial affairs are in order. I have a will, I've appointed the executor, and she has all the various contact and account information.

- because I've done my job, paid my dues and done right by everyone else, now it's time to do right by me.

- because I don't take any sort of medication and feel young enough to still have something to offer.

- because I still have a lot of "piss and vinegar" left in me.

Because I'm too damned young to be old.
I refuse to sit on the sidelines and knit. (Nothing wrong with knitting, I do it from time to time. Just not as a permanent retirement pastime.) I refuse to let my various aches and pains stand in the way of my adventures. Because to do so, to give it all up and sit on the sidelines, means dying a slow death.

And that's why I'm devoting the next 20 years to as much adventure as this weathered body can handle. Part of that adventure involves buying a motor home and cruising the countryside, visiting states I've never been to and exploring my own country.

I want to sip a fine Cabernet from a crystal glass by sunset in Napa Valley. I want to go camping in Alaska and watch the Northern Lights by the light of a campfire. I want to experience the majesty of Mt. Rushmore up close and personal. And I want to crack lobster in Maine like the "Maineiacs" do.

We'll travel overseas. England in spring is on my bucket list. Visions of rose-covered cottages, tiny villages and lambs frolicking across verdant pastures have danced in my head for the past 30 years. A European river cruise is on the adventure menu, as are Russia, Italy and Ecuador. Maybe even Turkey.

Then it's back to buy a piece of land and build a country cottage. Something that looks like it belongs in the country, not a lump of brick and mortar transplanted from the city. A house that's painted a soft pastel. Maybe green, or blue or yellow with black shutters. A country house with a white picket fence to support billowing antique roses.

We'll grow flowers and crops and raise chickens. It will involve hard work, and I might do it slower than younger folks, but I'll still do it. (Have you ever raised chickens? Talk about adventure…)

And the Harley will be our constant companion.

My cardiologist is pissed at me.
He became almost belligerent during my last visit as he insisted motorcycling would be my downfall. This, as he stubbornly tried to force me on blood thinners and statins using his strongest fear tactics. Turns out, he used to have a Harley, and his wife made him get rid of it. "For the children," she said.

I told him this: "I can either sit in a corner taking your blood thinners, afraid of my every movement, or I can live the adventure life's supposed to be. Either way, when it's my time to go, it's my time to go. I'll be damned if I die your way."

Now get out of my way, doc — I have places to go and people to see. On the back of a Harley.

Like a Fine Wine We Get Better with Age

By Michelle Monet

"Some people are old at 18, and some are young at 90...Time is a concept that humans created."

Yoko Ono

My boyfriend and I went to a concert last night. The band members were not youngsters. The lead singer was a dynamic performer who seemed to be at the top of his game. I loved to see it. He might have been in his late forties.

At the next table there were two talkative guys—one was an interesting musician/drummer. He was in his late fifties like me. We seemed to have a lot in common. (Both older yet bolder farts?)

We talked about entertainers who never retire but seem to get better with age.

He said, "I really do think that—like a fine wine, most musicians get better with time."

Hmm... *Most? Get better?* That's a cool statement.

I know *some* do, but I never thought *most* got better.

I know some have lost their voices and some probably should hang it up and retire— but many who don't retire seem to get better, more seasoned with time.

Here are a few famous people we both agreed were still *rockin' it* later in life. Many aren't showing many signs of slowing down, and might have even aged better like a fine wine in their later years:

Annie Lennox

Willie Nelson

Tony Bennett

Judy Collins

Steven Tyler

Brian Wilson

Rod Stewart

Barbra Streisand

Mick Jagger

Dick Van Dyke

Cloris Leachman

Betty White

I told him my goal was to write a musical, and that I have it partially done. He seemed excited for me.

I admitted, "Yes, I am older, grayer, chubbier, have more wrinkles and less stamina (at age 57) — but I also have more wisdom!"

He chuckled and nodded his head.

"Yes! Age is just a number. You go girl!"

I appreciated the cheerful encouragement.

There are days when I feel totally inspired. I believe I am better (and wiser) in my later years, which makes me encouraged about the aging process. (For instance, when I am rehearsing and coming up with new song ideas or new story ideas, or just getting new *AHAs*!)

Other days I feel weary because I know that my body has many obvious slowdowns from aging.

I prefer, though, to think that all my past experiences have gelled together to form who I am today and that I am better in every way. I love this affirmative statement, which I use often.

Every day in every way I am getting better and better !

How 'bout you? Do you feel you're getting better with time even if your physical body is showing signs of slowing down?

70s – Time to Slow Down?

By DB McNicol

No, not the 1970s, my 70s. I am already beyond that magic number by a couple of years. I've lived a lot, experienced a lot, lost a lot, gained a lot, but know there is more ahead. Every decade of my life has brought ups and downs, all accompanied by drama. The roller coaster of life -- personal and professional, private and public.

I am not my grandmother's 70s. I am not even my mother's 70s. I am mine — I am me, totally unique. Even as a Baby Boomer, my path has varied from many of my peers. I married young, had children young, worked full-time (sometimes two jobs), divorced young, remarried, another child, divorced again.

I was in my late 30s when I discovered a career and over the next thirty years I worked hard to move from a data entry operator to VP of Client Services. No college degree, raising children, surviving abusive marriages, but I still found my niche. Something I excelled at. There weren't many women working with computers, and it took many job changes to move up the ladder, but they were, for the most part, wonderful years.

I never minded aging, not turning 30, 40, or even 50. These are often milestone years, as is turning 60. For me, turning 60 meant I qualified for Social Security as a widow, having lost my soulmate two years earlier. It was the start of a grand adventure. Actually, it was my second grand adventure, the first being my solo motorcycle rides around the country, riding through 42 states and across 27,000 miles.

But on to 60 when I sold my house and everything else, bought a used Class C motorhome with a small trailer for my motorcycle and headed out to travel full-time. I was in Gillette, WY, when I met my current husband — also widowed, a full-time RVer and a motorcyclist. Fate, right? A year later in 2009 we married, and the adventures didn't slow down. It's true…age is just a number.

Over the last ten years we have traveled the country by RV through all 48 states and cruised to both Hawaii and Alaska. My husband helped me ride my motorcycle through the last six continental states, then we moved to Ecuador for two years, cruised multiple times, bought land and semi-developed it, bought a house and sold said land.

The adventure still continues. In addition, I published several mystery books, one romance, a couple of children's books, and had short stories published in anthology books.

Ah, yes, life has been good. But we have also lost several family members, too many friends (some way too young), and battled health issues. Life can rub your nose in your mortality. We're all going to die; we just don't know when.

I may be over 70 now and I may have slowed down from my 20s and 30s, but I don't intend to live quietly.

Unlock Your Bias – Old and Grey but We Still Rock

I may creak and click but I ain't done yet.

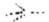

By Caroline de Braganza

I tuned in to the BBC World Service on Sunday afternoon. (No, not a church service — a radio station. It's been around since 1932 and still going strong. Radio never ages and will never die.)

Anyway, I caught an interview with Ashton Applewhite discussing her book *This Chair Rocks: A Manifesto against Ageism*. I'm dying to buy it (not THAT sort of dying) but will have to wait awhile. What she said resonated with me.

Bias in the Workplace

Her words took me back to four years ago when I retired *against my will*; I'd reached my sell-by age of 65, after which we are considered too old to be of any benefit to an employer. And our labor law in South Africa allows it, so I couldn't fight back against the discrimination.

Applewhite commented that many people are ashamed of being older. I'm not one of them, though I'm angry and frustrated that increased life expectancy hasn't yet been factored into employment practices.

Finding even a part-time job was out of the question. Believe me, I tried.

But for me it was a blessing as I turned my hand to writing, putting pen to paper and arthritic fingers to the keyboard.

The Blame Game

Shortly after *"retiring"* I joined a global online community that Coca Cola ran. It provided a rare occasion where my age was an advantage as they wanted broad representation of age groups and nationalities — I qualified!

I entered into a lively online debate with a young lady from India who said old people should quit their jobs to give room to the unemployed youth who can't get jobs. The implication was that we're in the way.

That's another point Applewhite covers in her book. We don't take jobs from others. When the labor market grows, employment opportunities grow for *all* age groups.

My final words to the young lady in India were that, following her logic, people with homes should move out so that the homeless can move in.* That put an end to that.

Self-discrimination

It's tragic that as we age, many of us buy into the belief that we're no longer useful, a belief driven by the bigotry embedded in the brands bashing us into submission.

They persuade us we'll feel much better about ourselves if we just cover up.

I have never bought into that philosophy. Ever. After all, age is a state of mind.

"You can't stop getting older, but you can stop growing old," says Marisa Peer, therapist, best-selling author and motivational speaker. We can't stop our biological clock. But we can keep our brains and bodies fit.

I remember a comment from a young writer from the UK on *Medium* in the early stages of my writing. He said I was nothing like his grandparents and thanked me for giving him an alternative way of looking at old people.

In the UK, BBC documentary-maker Tim Samuels set out in 2007 to make a film about how badly the elderly are treated in Britain.

Pensioners Pack a Punch
Samuels decided to form a band with the lonely old people he found in care homes, tower blocks and bingo halls. He wanted to give the elderly a voice.

What emerged was a mind-blowing cover version of The Who's "*My Generation*" recorded in the Beatles' old studio at Abbey Road. Forty people with no musical background got together to belt out the song.

Their video went to #1 on YouTube and #26 on the UK Singles Charts. They were a global sensation. Media from 50 countries wanted to interview them and they traveled to LA to appear on a chat show with George Clooney.

And for an encore, they performed the Beastie Boys' "*Fight For Your Right*" at *Britain's Got Talent* in 2012. (You can sense the prejudice when they first appear on stage fading as the judges and audience get in the groove.)

We still rock — and tango.

Let me assure you I have deep compassion for those without shelter anywhere in the world. The solution is to build more houses and ban real estate conglomerates. But that's another story.

PART FOUR: Transitions

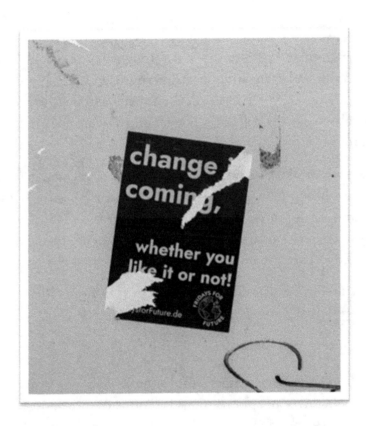

Find Your Superpowers After 50

By Ingrid L. Williams

Congratulations! You made it through the minefield that is youth and early adulthood. Intermingled with all the good times, delightful discoveries, achievements and joys, there were also false starts, dead ends, frenemies and unwelcome life lessons galore.

Guess what? Now it's time to move on to the next station on this journey through life. The great thing about this phase is that you are far from unprepared. In fact, you finally have advantages you may not even be aware of. Embrace them! And use them to make the second part of your life far better than the first one.

There are many gifts that time bestows upon those of us over 50 that are actually super tools for better life quality.

Here are some of the best:

You Don't Care What Other People Think

Boohooing over people who dislike you is over. You just avoid those folks and don't even think about them. You will walk through fire for what you believe in because you can't be asked to not be yourself. There is just no pay-off big enough or meaningful enough to carry on with faking this or that. It's incredibly ok to not be in agreement with everyone, even the people you love or respect. Other people's opinions no longer govern or dictate how you live.

You Dare
You know that the worst thing that could happen is not the end of the world. And even if it is, you will survive that, too.

You Have Learned To Enjoy Your Own Company.
You may even discover that you crave alone time. Then you begin to require it. Hell, sometimes your own company is about all you can stand.

You Are No Longer In The Beauty Pageant
Think of all the hours you spent in your more youthful days desperately seeking that one magical shade of lipstick or the perfect split skirt that would reveal just enough thigh to make you look enticing, but not easy. Remember how vital it seemed to look as amazing as possible at practically every hour of the day in order to satisfy "the gaze?" And the competition was grim, mean-spirited and relentless.

Well, now you are off the radar screen of everyone, male or female, under 50. This means you can focus on the things you discovered are actually important. The freedom of this cannot be underestimated.

You Know What's Actually Important
Your earlier days were spent living like a pinball inside a brightly lit machine full of noise where you were batted around aimlessly for reasons you could never quite sort out. But you were actually

the driver of that situation because it was all about your process of trying on different goals, lifestyles, relationships, personas and endless variations of everything else. Which seemed important at the time. That you now laugh about.

You thought you needed a PR-generating career, a beach house in Miami, an Italian sports car and the world at your feet. Now you know all you truly need is a peaceful, secluded room with a secure lock, your private blanket, a glass of wine and a good book.

You Have A Highly Developed Bullshit Meter

Thanks to all the years of stumbling, fumbling and fool's gold stampedes, your eyes are wide open, and your palate is officially jaded. Whether it is political promises, infomercials, cosmetics, the latest fad, weight loss programs or slick life-hacking apps, your pulse simply refuses to rise in excitement. You have seen snake oil come and snake oil go. F*ck snake oil.

You Realize You Are Not Immortal And The Clock Is Ticking

This means you are forced to decide what your personal agenda on this planet really is and how badly you actually want it. If you are not willing to make it a priority and sacrifice for it, it falls off the list in favor of the things you actually burn for.

Whether your dream is to bring clean water to the remote villages of a foreign country, to establish an animal rescue shelter in your county or finally bake the perfect souffle, you begin to realize it is just about time to get on with putting that plan into action. If it is ever going to happen. You recognize that you have been put on notice.

Your Hustle Is Deep

You remember that time before the internet when you just had to be resourceful. You know there is more than one way to skin a cat — and thoroughly. You don't expect instant results or feel that the world owes you a living and all the avocado toast you desire, so you don't deal in magical thinking. You know that defeat is usually a speed bump, not a roadblock. You show up willing to do the work you know is necessary to get what you want, and then some. You plunge forward because you know that there is really no other option, even if you might have to go sideways temporarily. But just until you figure it out. Which you will.

You Have Learned When To Walk Away And Not Bother

It takes years of entering conversations that were never going to lead to anyplace good before you recognize when you are teetering on the edge of falling into one of them again and pull yourself back from the brink.

You Know "Tomorrow Is Another Day"

If you have gotten this far in life with any measure of success, Scarlett O'Hara is pretty much your spirit animal by now. So, her final line in *Gone With The Wind* resonates with you. You really get it. You understand the sinking of her world-weary shoulders, her frantic, tearful desperation dwindling down to wistful longing, her frank recognition that the battle of the moment is over and that she will have to withdraw from the field. For the day, anyway. She has hardly given up, but it's time for a little gathering in and reflection before resuming the war.

Like Scarlett, you have learned to accept that setbacks are inevitable, but that you are resilient. That there will be something to carry on for or with. At some of the roughest moments in life, you sometimes need to put the burden down and just take a nap or something before you resume the struggle. Getting that lesson down means you have figured out when to pause for a moment and hit the reset button.

Five Tips for a Happy Midlife Career Exit

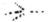

By Kathleen Cardwell

At 53 years old, I was coasting along in my career of three decades in the corporate world and in higher education. The mileage was there in my graying hair and in my laugh lines. I had become seasoned with a calm demeanor, a few life lessons, and a quiet self-confidence. I was more than comfortable being that vintage car on the corner of the lot, squeezed in between the newer models.

But slowly, I realized it was time for me to go. Years of leadership changes and silly office dramas had started to wear me down. Even worse was the telltale sign: zero motivation and passion for my work.

The spark was gone, and it wasn't coming back.

I knew submitting my letter of resignation was the point of no return. Determined to be my professional and thorough self, I also knew I had to be present in each moment and soak it all in. After all, I was walking (*skipping, actually*) away from a respectable salary and incredible benefits. Recruiters weren't knocking on my door. I didn't have a new job to go to. Besides a meager paycheck from adjunct teaching, my income and my life were about to go topsy-turvy.

These five unexpected strategies ultimately held me together through the end and into a new beginning:

Tie Up All The Loose Ends

I created a countdown journal where I could collect my daily thoughts and musings. I turned all of my projects over to people I knew would finish them to my standards. I collected samples of all my work and purged all the useless stuff, including every single cheesy professional development certificate from the human resources department. I thanked the facilities staff and the mailroom team for putting up with my messes and my indiscriminate rants. And yes, during that final team meeting, I pretended to like *that one person* for the last time.

During this initial phase, I also started to appreciate the importance of finding grace in every moment. From the dreaded good-byes to the awkward going-away party, I was determined to be my best genuine self, to depart on a good, happy note.

Struggle Through A Deep-Dive Reality Check

I experienced days of self-doubt, days of indignant pride, and days of sadness. I would remind myself that I had earned this opportunity, this chance of a lifetime. But there were so many times when my heart felt heavy. I would stare into the mirror, asking those questions we're all destined to ask. Where did the time go? Why didn't I do this when I was younger?

Gavin was the chirpy investment advisor who was unfortunate enough to get my phone call about my latest life change. He told me, "Your retirement strategy isn't sustainable."

No sh*t. Do you mean if I quit contributing a boatload of money to my 401K it will wither away and I'll have no money for when I'm actually an old person? Good to know.

I obsessed with staying busy every hour of every day for the first few weeks after I quit. I stuck to my schedule of waking up early and exercising, followed by researching and planning what the next phase of my life would be. And yes, I got dressed every day as if I was going to work.

Channel Your Neglected Creative Outlets

I giggled like a child when I rediscovered my coveted sketch pad and pencils, my basket of embroidery projects, and the crossword puzzles in the Sunday paper. I returned to writing for the sheer sake of writing, an innate passion which had been sidelined for so long. It beckoned often, but I was too busy working for other people.

Redirecting my energy and reigniting my creative side were immensely important transitions for me. They allowed me to cleanse my persona and finally detach from my former life. I became open to ideas and possibilities.

Be Your Ridiculous, Funny Self

I was hell-bent on ensuring my grand exit did not include me lugging a box of office toys and worn file folders out the door. So, I deployed the Andy Dufresne method from the 1994 movie, *The Shawshank Redemption*. Andy (played by Tim Robbins) digs an escape tunnel in his cell. During his daily stroll in the prison yard, he discretely discards the leftover rocks through holes in the pockets of his pants.

For three weeks, I took things home a few items at a time, in my backpack or stuffed in the deep recesses of my purse. A framed photo, coffee mugs, my coveted rubber band ball. It took some ingenuity, cowardice, and covert maneuvers to get the big stuff out of my office. I stayed late after work to remove my two desk lamps and a small bookshelf in the dark of the night. I loaded spare shoes and my lumbar pillow in my gym bag. Plants were left in the kitchenette with "FREE!" signs attached to them.

No one was the wiser.

Search Your Soul, Then Trust Your Gut
Within the first two months of my intentional unemployment, my husband said, "You won't have any trouble finding another job with your experience."

He was wrong. I was drowning in rejection emails. As a fifty-something Baby Boomer with proven success, how was I no longer relevant anywhere or to anyone? More than once I panicked, feeling foolish, impetuous, and irresponsible. But I followed my gut and focused on what I knew was right for me, which was not to return to the full-time rat race.

I also allowed myself to remember the feeling of that last day. It was a freeing of my spirit and the chill of the unknown, wrapped up in a ball of excitement and fear.

Happily, I didn't feel old. I felt alive.

What's Next?

Eight months have passed, and I have never, ever, regretted my decision. I'm working a part-time job to help pay the bills, and it has been incredibly humbling to learn what I can live without. I'm also venturing into the world of freelance writing and editing, to see where it takes me. I'm truer to myself now than I have ever been.

I know that I have more years behind me than I do in front of me. The occasional days of doubt still linger. But here's the kicker. I now get to begin each day deciding who and what is going to get the best of all I have to offer.

It's about time.

Retirement

By Greg Hopkins

For 40 years you're the star of "This is Me at Work!" When the show ends, so does the character you've become. How you deal with the obliteration of this role sets the course for the rest of your life.

My final moments at work were unremarkable. There was no applause or tearful goodbyes. Just another ordinary, humdrum day. Except, this time, when the office door closed behind me, it was over for good.

I remember walking to my car, carrying odds and ends from my desk, and feeling the cumulative weight of 40 years in the workforce cloaking me with disappointment and disbelief. *This was it? Really?*

Work never did deliver on the promise that, someday, *I'll strike it rich!* The carrot, dangling in front of me all those years, turned out to be plastic. I felt every bit the donkey who had plodded after the damn thing. Now what the hell was I supposed to do?

Far from sitting on a porch sipping a glass of tea, or walking on endless beaches, the onset of retirement is more like being marched to a cliff and forced to jump.

In my case, I figured as long as I was jumping, let's jump. My wife and I packed up and moved to Uruguay two weeks after my last day of work. The shock of retirement was overshadowed by the even greater upheaval of leaving everything I'd known. Getting the house cleared out, wrapping things up, and leaving town was a harrowing, traumatizing ordeal. But I'm grateful that, with ample encouragement from my wife, things played out this way. I had a definite ending and a new beginning, on my own terms.

In my three years living in Uruguay, I actually walked my share of beaches and occasionally sipped tea on a porch. But the past intruded on my days. Feelings of unfinished business, regrets, and a longing for the elixir of success haunted me. I was unmistakably navigating through the stages of grief.

The thing about something ending — a death — is the loss of not only the end of what was, it's also the end of everything that could have been. All the things that were hoped for now can never be.

Truth be told, I didn't bear the load of daily work well. I tended to crumble under pressure. Even when I delivered the goods, I was often sweating bullets. I lashed out at people. I dropped a lot of balls. I failed, often and egregiously.

It wasn't supposed to turn out like that. Work was supposed to be a redemption and exoneration. A chance to triumph. I had my moments in the spotlight. Transient as these were, they existed. To paraphrase Ken Wilber, nobody's smart enough to fail all the time. But, somehow, the fuck ups, shortcomings and train wrecks cast a longer shadow than the laughter, high-fives and acceptance speeches.

I wrote a lot of letters in my head apologizing to former coworkers and asking their forgiveness. In the end, none of these were sent. The anxious, disturbing memories that woke me up at night were more than likely long forgotten in the minds of others, and over-exaggerated in mine. And, practically speaking, I'd lost touch with nearly everyone from past employment.

In the end, it was me who needed to forgive myself and let go of the past. It's taken time, but I have to say it's coming along. It was difficult to face up to the stinging truth that nobody on the planet gives a *flying fuck* about what I did, and didn't do, over the course of 79,000 cumulative hours on the clock.

But here's the good thing. Nothing, and nobody at all, is holding me back from moving on.

Acceptance feels oddly open-ended. But more and more, the notion of just *being* makes sense to me. It has something to do with knowing that life is infinitely vaster and more intelligent than anything my localized identity, with its yammering brain, could cook up. I feel called to stop trying to run and simply allow life to express through me.

Looking back, I can see how the constant, restless drive to accomplish something, to succeed, was driven by an undercurrent of greed and fear, fueled by the belief that we're on our own in the jungle of life. I'm glad to let that story go.

The next phase of my life, which could be 30 years long, promises to yield wonderful surprises I could never dream of. It already has, and things are just getting started. I'm learning, slowly, to trust.

How to Age Well and Have Your Best Later Life

It's time to celebrate the gift of aging.

By Zoe Berry

Aging is a part of life. As a nurse, I've cared for the aging and dying. I'm now assisting my 90+ year-old mother in her final years and, since my recent retirement from a 40-year healthcare career, I'm learning how to manage my own aging. But what do we mean by aging?

It is the process of getting older, in which we will face physical, psychological and social changes. Aging starts almost from the moment we are born, but at this stage, it's a cause for celebration. We watch and marvel at how babies develop and transform in what seems like a blink of an eye.

But at some point, our attitude toward aging changes and for many, it becomes a cause for concern. That's understandable; aging, or more specifically being "aged," is often associated with increasing frailty, loss of independence, disability and dementia. But does it need to be this way?

Naturally, each of us experiences the aging of our bodies in our own way and in our own time. And there are, of course, many differing and sometimes contradictory views toward aging. What do I mean by that?

Alternative Views Toward Aging

There is an increasing number of inspiring images of older women featured in the media, and influential women in their forties and fifties often speak positively about their awareness of the onset of physical changes as they age.

As 52-year-old TV presenter Davina McCall said, *"We may have a few more wrinkles now, but with that comes life experience."*

At the same time, there are younger women, some in their teenage years, seeking cosmetic procedures to delay what they perceive as the negative physical effects of time passing.

Recently I saw a newspaper article promoting a new book about an anti-aging program designed to help you "look and feel younger" and I wondered what that might mean. Have we stopped to think about what might be more important, to look younger or to *feel* younger?

I should say that, as a former nurse, I am an advocate for anyone, at any age, taking positive steps to optimize their health, and as an older person I want to look and feel my best. But does that mean I want to look and feel younger? After all, for many people, youth and middle age may not have been that great, for whatever reason. There are good things about not being the same person you were in your younger days: all those mistakes and poor decisions, the fashion embarrassments, and the highly questionable hairstyles!

But why should we be *anti*-aging? Isn't that ageist, and at the very least, doesn't that sound unnecessarily negative?

The Case For Being Anti-"Anti-Aging"

A child born today has a higher chance of living to over 105 years than in any previous generation; that means many more old people in the future. So, shouldn't we be redefining and reviewing our attitudes towards old age?

Ask yourself, is being told you look younger than your age a compliment? If so, why? And how young should any older person aspire to look and feel? If I'm 60, do I want to look 50 or 45? If I'm 80 do I want to look 70? Why? What would that "achievement" mean?

Not so long ago, young people would attempt to look older because, in many cases, it was older people who held positions of power. That isn't true anymore. Just look around at the many younger business leaders in the tech industry, for example.

Now it is older people who have to compete with and emulate the young. Recently I came across the term "juvenescence", which is the state of being youthful or "growing young." That concept places undue pressure on the older person and I suggest that the whole idea of *"anti-aging" is nothing more than a marketing technique that attempts to sell us everlasting youth!*

A Positive Approach To Aging

How we look and how we age biologically is, to a great extent, down to genetics but also a result of some decisions and actions we took in our younger years. For example, how many of us growing up in the 1960s would have taken the precaution to slather ourselves in sunscreen as we roasted on the beach?

In other words, aside from cosmetic cover-ups, dental work and good aesthetic procedures, we may not have much choice about how we look as we age.

As for "feeling young," it's not at all uncommon for older people to describe how they just don't feel their age. Or the mild shock they experience when they look in the mirror and see a face that just doesn't seem to reflect the age they feel.

Age is just a number. Old age creeps up on us all but there is probably a particular age at which you will feel old. For the author Diana Athill, who died in 2019 at the age of 100, old age started at 71. In her book, "*Somewhere Towards The End*," she wrote:

"All through my sixties, I felt I was still within hailing distance of middle age... but my seventy-first did change it. Being 'over seventy' is being old: suddenly I was aground on that fact and saw that the time had come to size it up."

Diana decided to retire at 75.

Not so long ago, we used to characterize our lives as having three distinct stages: education, career and retirement. With lengthening lifespans and changing models of employment there is now the opportunity to view life as having many stages, career changes and breaks.

Young people today are facing a world in which *flexibility, adaptability and life-long learning* are important attributes. Maybe *these* are the youthful qualities that we elders need to emulate, so we are better equipped to steer our way through the inevitable changes we will face as we age.

It's Not Too Late To Make Plans

I believe we should live in the present to appreciate life as it unfolds, rather than worrying about an uncertain future. However, in my experience both personally and professionally, I have seen the difference a little planning ahead can make to the quality of life as we age. Planning positive changes, big and small, such as keeping fit and eating more healthily, and considering what sort of housing might best suit us in the future, can be key factors to living well for longer.

Long-life was once seen as a curse but we should celebrate aging as a gift, a gift of time. It is a joyous time to be alive.

And the Years Have Flown Away Like the Leaves on a Mid-October Day

A talk with my elderly neighbor.

By Julia E. Hubbel

Outside the living room window, the cottonwood leaves are tossed by the late afternoon breeze, their usual bright yellow darkened by a harsh early frost. Just after I got home from Mongolia, our usually 65-ish October days were briefly blasted by a fall storm that dragged our temperatures down 60 plus degrees in the space of barely a day, an all-time record. What has fallen isn't gold. It's dusky brown. Still, the leaves swirl prettily in the breeze as Emma (not her real name) and I watch. My house is just across the street, the aspens shattering a trail of brown coins over the grass.

Emma is watching the last of her years, in effect. Her home of the last fifty years is wide open. People have been tromping through all day picking through the memories and touchstones of her long life. When she and her husband moved in, I was just arriving in Colorado, all excited and dewy-eyed, as so many others are doing right now.

Each item handled by a stranger carries the weight of six decades of love, kids, struggles, pain and happiness. The dresser, ten dollars, which had housed clothing lovingly folded and tucked away. Kid's toys and remembrances. The dishes that served a family for years. Now, pennies for memories. She can't watch. What she wants to keep is all jammed into a back bedroom, where she is, waiting for the march of strangers carrying the evidence of her long life away from her forever to Just. End. Already.

Emma's 88. Her husband died suddenly of a brain aneurysm two years ago. That was her hard freeze.

The World Health Organization reports that on average, women live six to eight years longer than men. Right at the most vulnerable times of their lives, they're alone.

Since then she's been saddled with this big, rambling house, and all the care and demands that such a place puts on her stooped shoulders. Stripped of her moral and emotional support, and her lifetime helper, she was consumed by the house and its endless repairs.

The kids have been great. From the beginning they've assisted, from hiring my lawn guy to trim the huge, stately trees that are a hallmark of this block to helping her make some final decisions about where to land. In this regard, Emma has effectively hit the jackpot. This past summer, while I was away in Canada, one daughter came across a place north of here that was about to open. They cater to elders, and they needed an activities director. One thing led to another, and Emma had a place. Her daughter has a job, right on site. Perfect.

There are few more ideal situations, in addition to the fact that this place is near her family up north, which means they can avoid the awful traffic. She will see them more often, because, as she said, they're great kids.

I dragged Emma out of her bedroom where she was hiding from the estate sale. We haven't talked a lot, but I've been very aware of her situation. She was happy for a familiar face, not another stranger digging around for more bargains in what was once her castle, her Safe Place. Now the wind blew leaves into the empty kitchen from the spacious back yard, which, much like mine, is lined with shade trees. The evening chill had begun to touch the living room as the trickle of folks and curious neighbors dwindled.

Her eyes were tired, but she was committed. "It's time," she said. "The house is too much."

It's also an echo chamber for a marriage of 61 years. Every room is a whisper or a shout, just as every item that still sits for sale on the many tables bears witness to a long life. Trinkets gathered from travels, gifts given, received and cherished.

Emma told me about her new place. The exercise room, the food, the activities. Most of all, her daughter would be there. Her eyes lit up. That would make it a Safe Place, and we both knew it. I am delighted for her.

Most of us don't get that special sauce of a family member who could run point, keep an eye out, and stay close once we've given up the comfort of a familiar place. We should all be so lucky. My other neighbor, whose husband died suddenly some years ago, had to do the same thing. It was a harder experience.

The leaves twirled like fairies. Life goes on. Things die, are born. Neither of us would be here next fall to see these trees, these breezes. Emma's moving just in time for Thanksgiving. She won't have to suffer through another holiday season with sixty years of dinners and gifts and laughter and presents following her around the place like an aging dog.

As she spoke, I considered. She knows I'm moving; she's seen the boxes and the packing and the preparations. We both know how hard it is to let go of the familiar. But Emma has lost more, the history of her long marriage. She now needs to fill that chasm with friends and activity. The move is right, albeit scary.

My options are different. As Emma's life is slowing down, mine is speeding up. But in perhaps twenty or so years, I may well be faced with the same imminent decisions. Twenty years aren't that many. After all, I could see the look on Emma's face as we watched the leaves. It mirrored mine.

My god. Sixty-one years. Where on earth did it all go? How did I get here so fast?

I don't have family or kids. My move is going to be motivated by the need, in part, to get to a place, make friends and establish my own network long before I really need it. I've got time, Emma doesn't. But Emma has family, and I don't. I have to make one. I can, but it takes time and commitment.

The phone rang. It's on the wall and has a long, curled cord. Of course it does. It was Meg, her best friend. Emma has a dinner date tonight. Women like us need dinner dates; Emma perhaps more than I do. For now.

Emma is in good and loving hands. That's not always the case for elders. We all need advocates and friends and family who really do look out for us, as Emma's kids do for her. For as she and I watched, with pleasure, the leaves trace a do-si-do on my driveway and across her lawn, we were also watching the passage of time in both our lives.

This is our last fall here. Forever.

For me the words fall with a terrible finality. I will leave behind 50 years, my entire adult life, in Denver. I am off to parts unknown.

Emma is leaving behind 61 years of memories, to parts better known, peopled with family and the comfort of familiar faces.

Two aging women, facing an uncertain future.

The leaves lifted, waved, and whisked down the street, as quickly as all the years of our long lives.

PART FIVE: An Ounce of Wisdom

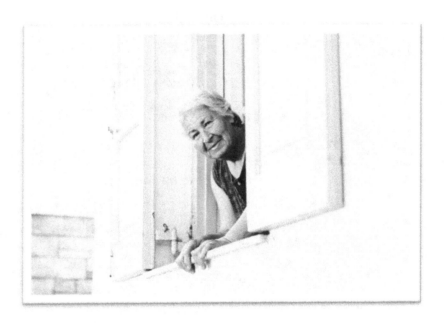

What Matters
A Poem of New-found Wisdom

By Dennett

Years dwindle,

a countdown in reverse —

many scratch Bucket Lists

of all not done to be done.

Not I —

No lists of incomplete dreams,

not because I have none

but because they

no longer matter —

I have what I need,

the rest is waste —

a lesson of age and

maybe, wisdom.

Resting in "Being" After a Lifetime of "Doing"

Overcoming the need to be productive, to be worthy

By Beth Bruno

We live in a world where productivity is god. If you are a functioning adult, you are expected to do things that prove you are valuable to society. You must pull your load, make a living, contribute. We derive our sense of self-worth from our doing, because that is what we are taught from the time we are in school.

So, what happens when we come to a place in our lives where we feel like we are no longer a contributing member of society? How do we make the transition from "doer" to simply resting in being?

This is a question that my mother has been grappling with lately. At 80 years old she is dealing with an illness that has taken a lot of her strength. While she is still able to do things for herself, she is unable to care for those around her the way she once did, and her social activities have been curtailed.

Mom is an amazing woman. She has raised three great kids, lavishing love and encouragement on all of us. She has been a tremendous influence on her many grandchildren. She has run successful businesses as a female entrepreneur. She is a musician, a fiber artist, a gardener, and an interior designer.

As Mother is thinking about her life, she wonders "What now?" She feels like she is not much use anymore. She doesn't have the energy to do any of those things now. Much of what she invested herself in to create her identity has fallen away. And because we gain our sense of self from what we DO, it is difficult to change our ideas about that.

Resting in being is different than being busy and productive. It requires a level of trust that we have not learned to bring to our lives and our selves. It means we have to believe that we are worthy just because we have had the privilege to be alive on this planet. That we do not have to earn our right to be here. That we are enough.

When you are 80 years old, this can seem impossible.

When your life of activity and productivity diminishes, it feels like you are diminished, too. We have spent a lifetime evaluating, judging and assessing whether we are doing enough, getting it right, a value to others. We have a voice in our head that keeps up a constant monologue about our worth. This voice is not usually very friendly.

So, of course, when we are no longer able to do what we could once do — those things we thought were necessary to justify our existence — we can feel like we are careening off a ledge into the vast nothingness.

We spend our lives trapped in our egoic thinking that we are what we accomplish, our talents, our personality, our thinking. What we are missing is that we have a being within us that rests in the midst of all of that and most of us go an entire lifetime without even realizing it is there. That being is the part of us that is connected to spirit, the part that has no fear, no anxiety, no shame.

Simply resting in being human means dropping down into ourselves and connecting with our pure self — "the one who knows." The one who understands that your life is valuable just because you exist here. Now you have time to be still and connect with that part of you that has been neglected. As the busy-ness diminishes, it makes room for the "being" to expand.

Now, there is time to do something that very few of us ever learn to do — live in the moment. Settle into each moment as it comes, and really pay attention. Noticing the way the light dances across the floor when the sun streams in the windows. Looking out and seeing the view — really seeing it. Paying attention to the warmth of a soft blanket, the deliciousness of a lemony dessert, the love in someone's eyes.

Simply being means being present to life as it presents itself each moment, without the shadow of worry for the future. This moment, and this, and then this. And practicing gratitude for all of it. For what is now, for what has been.

There is time to read all the books you never had time to read in all your busy-ness. You can watch TV without guilt. You can sit on your porch when the weather is nice and drink your tea and read the paper. No hurry, no worry. You can relish all you have accomplished in this life. You can be proud of the legacy of love you have built for your family and friends. You can remind yourself that it is enough. More than enough.

Back in the day, Mom was a mean fisherman. She had a sense for where the fish were hiding, deep at the bottom of the river. She also knew exactly where the anchor was that she and my stepdad lost at the bottom of that river. He went out and looked for it every day for a week. After his failed attempts, Mom said she knew where it was. They went back out in the boat the next day and mom pointed to the spot. It was a big, wide river. But she found that anchor. Mom has always had a way of seeing that few possess.

Learning to rest in being is a lot like that. We have to reach down in the murky depths, seeing what is there, though it is clouded over by the churning muddy water of "doing." When we begin to rest in being, the mud begins to settle. Then we can see what was there all along. Our human worth resides solely in our being.

How Terribly Not Strange To Be (Almost) Seventy

By Paul Hossfield

I've thought about this before. In fact, I wrote about it in September of 2018. At that time, I was 68 and had more than a year to go. Rather than The Beatles' "*When I'm Sixty-four,*" I thought about the album "*Bookends,*" a studio album by Simon and Garfunkel released in April of 1968, when I was 18. Bookends contains the song "*Old Friends,*" which in turn contains the haunting line, "*how terribly strange to be seventy.*"

At eighteen I could not imagine being seventy. I was still in love with my first serious girlfriend in an all-encompassing way that happens with teenagers. Unfortunately, I was still a jerk at that age, as a result of which I was to experience my first serious breakup in a month or so, but of course I had no idea.

But seventy! I remember thinking, that's so *old*! Now it will be upon me in less than six months. I'm thinking my seventieth birthday will be *just another day.* Didn't the Beatles write a song with that title also?

Over this past year I put a new thing in my life, one which has proven so much fun that it's hard to believe: Membership in The Extraordinary Rendition Band (ERB), an activist street band. If this has taught me anything it's that putting a new thing in your life renews it. It's like a breath of air from a new country. A new thing can also upend your life, but be not afraid, new things are good. That thought is hardly original. Read a few self-helpie type articles and you are sure to run across it.

In my case, my new thing has kept me away from my long-established thing of Aikido. I'm down to about once a week, and I really need to get there at least twice a week in order for it to serve its purpose of keeping my body from becoming stiff. To do that I need at least *three* possible days, because stuff happens. Classes are available Monday, Wednesday, Thursday, and Saturday. Rhode Island Civic Chorale meets on Wednesday and ERB meets on Thursday. Since I only just got started with ERB and, more importantly, because it is so much fun, I'm putting that in the keeper column.

It will be sad to leave the Civic Chorale, especially because we have a dynamic new director, and our recent performance of G. F. Handel's oratorio *Messiah* was such an absolute, mind-blowing smash. I'll keep telling myself that it was a good performance to go out on. My memories of Rhode Island Civic Chorale will be suffused with beauty. One of my besties thinks I'm making a mistake, but I need to make the choice. Even at seventy life is about making choices.

One of the things I notice is that standing bothers me, whereas movement has the power to take the standing pain away, especially lateral hip movement. ERB involves such movement, especially when we get into our "coreo." Civic chorale is mostly a stand-there-and-sing choir. So there is another reason to put it on the chopping block. Gospel choirs are not like that, so I'm sticking with the Exult Gospel Choir. Exult does not have regular rehearsals. Instead, a series of rehearsals are scheduled in advance of each concert. Therefore, it does not regularly stand in the way of Aikido.

I continue to thank God that the increasingly worrisome pains are controllable and that I can continue to do all that I do. You don't know what the future will bring but right now seventy is looking like it will be a good year.

I am still getting everywhere by bicycle although I am not as *hardcore* as formerly. For example, tonight I faced a good hour-plus bike ride from home on a drizzly night with my baritone horn on my back.

I was grateful when my wife texted me and offered to come get me. Which reminds me of one more life circumstance for which I am overflowing with gratitude: that I have such a wonderful life partner. She is always there for me and continues to inspire me with all *she* does.

I Have Lived 80 Years But Have I Learned Anything?

By Warren Turner

Actually, I have found no sane way to avoid aging, so I am going to refine my eldership before I run completely out of time.

Once during a Q & A session at a political forum, a woman prefaced her question by saying "Astonishingly, I turned 80 last week." I now know exactly what she meant because I just did, too.

It is a cliché that we feel one age in our mind, but we are chronologically another. Or as the legendary pitcher Satchel Paige famously said, "How old would you be if you didn't know how old you were?"

Meanwhile there are mirrors, group photos, upgraded pains, and the nice, but sometimes a bit tongue-in-cheek, compliment: "You can't be 80! I'd have never guessed."

So, what now? I will call myself an "elder." I don't really seem to have much wisdom. I do have some, even though much of it seems to have come lately. Maybe one has to trade off: One gem for each new ache. So, here are a few I have accumulated:

Screw Guilt

Have you murdered someone?* No? Then forget all that junk from your past.

In 12-step programs, essential work is to "take a personal inventory" and then to let it go and move on. Not possible, you say? Then try to change the past. Talk about impossible.

Shame Is In The Eye Of The Experiencer

Sometimes it is natural to feel ashamed, but ask yourself, why?

Let's say, no one knows or ever will know about what you are ashamed of. So, try this: Stand in front of a mirror and repeat after me, Shame begone!

OK Is Just OK

A relentless TV commercial makes fun of people who are not perfect. "Just OK is not OK," but is that true?

Some things have to be almost exactly right but for most of what we do or are, OK is definitely enough.

Being In Control Is A Hopeless Quest

If you have ever been called a "control freak," sit down and ponder that accusation.

This wisdom came from my daughter. I was once half worrying and half grieving over someone's situation. When I told her how I was feeling, she simply said, "You can't control anything in life." A radical statement but simply true.

That's it for now but after writing this, I remember that "I know a lot of things because I have seen a lot of things." That phrase may be the best definition of elderhood. If you are anything like me, I bet you have much wisdom, too.

*If you have actually murdered someone, that is above my paygrade. Sorry.

New Love After Loss – A Valentine of Hope

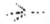

By Katharine Esty, PhD

I'm just back from a trip to Florida with my new love, Peter. We had a week of nice dinners and leisurely joys: looking at the ocean, talking, reading, and watching TV. Of course, it was an eighty-something-style holiday... slower and quieter than vacations at earlier ages. Peter used a wheelchair at the airport. I walked alone on the beach each morning because his walker doesn't work on sand. And we took a lot of naps. Sometimes two a day. But we felt so lucky and so happy to be together.

When my husband, John, died in 2015 it seemed to me I would never feel right again. Everything felt different and grey. My beloved husband of 59 years was gone. I was alone.

A year later, Michael, an elementary school classmate, got in touch with me and we went to lunch. I realized how lonely I had been and how glad I was for his company. But after a few months, I realized I didn't really like spending time with him. He didn't talk much or laugh much. He was no fix for my loneliness. So, I stopped seeing him.

At every age, some relationships just don't work out and we need to employ our break-up skills. (It wasn't all that easy.)

As another year passed, Peter, who was in my small support group, became my regular dinner companion. We spent more and more time together, gradually becoming a couple. Peter and I had lots to talk about. I felt safe.

Looking back, I was ready for a new love. I'll never stop missing John, but I let go of the acute grief and the numbness of the previous two years. I could let myself take the risk of loving.

I learned about loss, grieving, letting go, and loving again not only from my own experience but also much from the 128 people in their eighties who I interviewed for my book, *Eightysomethings: A Practical Guide to Letting Go, Aging Well, and Finding Unexpected Happiness* (Skyhorse, 2019).

By age 80, we have all experienced loss. Many of us have lost our spouse. All of us have lost friends. Some unlucky ones have lost a child. We've lost numerous pets. And we all know that to love again is risky. Several people told me they refused to get a new dog because the thought of losing another dog was just too painful.

To be ready to take the risk of new love, I've learned you need to grieve your losses one by one. One woman I interviewed told me that whenever a friend died, she 'd take what she called a 'private retreat' for an hour or so. She'd fully remember her friend, feel her sadness and think about attributes of her friend that she would try to incorporate into her own life going forward.

Grieving is, of course, an individual matter. There is no set timetable — it can take months or many years. But when the time is right, and you've grieved enough, for now anyway, you'll let go. And return to life and love.

Once we have passed the acute grieving stage, we will probably be ready to love again, to give fully — and it doesn't have to be romantic love. Get a new pet, make a new close friend, spend more time with a grandchild, or find a new companion or partner. Experience, once again, the pleasure of loving. Know again that the greatest pleasure in life is loving another. It is not being loved by someone else. Many of us don't learn this truth until late in life.

In case you're wondering, most eighty-somethings usually don't marry their new romantic loves. Life is way too complicated by children, finances, property, and health issues. And we relax as we see that new loves do not take the place of earlier loves. They are not in competition for the same space.

Peter and I keep separate apartments though we spend much time together. We have lots of photos of our spouses and children on our walls and we both wear our wedding rings. But for now, we are here for each other, and we are grateful.

Love is essential at every stage of life. As humans, we're adaptable and creative in where and how we find new love. Even in the most dire of experiences, we can love. It is like the surprising flower that valiantly emerges from a pile of rocks. We can all, at every age, learn to grieve, let go, and love again.

Life at 102

By Nancy Peckenham

My mother turned 102 on Sunday. She arrived at her party dressed in a powder blue wool jacket, her face animated by a smile she could not control. She didn't even try.

She basked in the glory of the day, aware that she had made it to another milestone, unlike any family member before. With a small group of friends and family gathered around her, she agreed that she was getting "kind of old."

What's it like to be 102? As in all of life, much depends on your state of mind. I see my mother daily and can report that she takes pleasure in each new day.

"Having a sense of humor is key to old age," she announced after eating cake at her party. "And never hold a grudge."

Her eyesight has almost completely failed but she sees sunshine when she looks out the window, even when it is rain. It used to bother me when I was younger that my mother rarely acknowledged any emotion that wasn't upbeat. Now I see that her positivity allows her to savor life while it boosts the spirits of her elderly neighbors in the assisted living home. I find peace myself when I follow her lead.

My mother made up her mind decades ago that she would never complain. She doesn't even grimace when she stands up, despite the back pain from three compacted vertebrae.

"What difference would it make if I talk about my aches and pains? No one listens anyway," she often says with a chuckle.

Her short-term memory loss can be another blessing. She may feel a shooting pain from time-to-time but when she is settled in a comfortable chair or talking to friends, she doesn't remember that she ever had any discomfort.

My mother isn't looking for sympathy. Having someone to talk to is at the top of her list. The social skills she learned in college back in the 1930s make it easy for her to break the ice with strangers. They are drawn to this tiny little lady who puts two hands on the top of her walker and bends her head back to look into their eyes. Who could walk away without greeting her in return?

Longevity doesn't just come from a positive attitude, however. If it did, we wouldn't lose good folks at a younger age.

Genetics play a role and the ones you get are often the luck of the draw. My mother had three sisters, one died at age 66, another at 72 and the third in her mid-80s. It's hard to say what genetic factors are at play in mother's long life. Scientists have only begun to explore the relationship between genes and health. It's an exciting field but one with miles of work to be done.

Another factor in my mother's longevity is the amount of physical activity she took on later in life. In her 60s, she threw herself into gardening, tending a huge perennial flower garden into her mid-80s. She never asked for help to lug around soil or dig up roots. Being on her hands and knees seemed to give her a boost.

Once she moved into an apartment, walking became her activity of choice. All year round she would travel on foot, up and down hills and around town. Drivers occasionally stopped their cars to offer her a ride. She always declined.

As a result, when my mother fell at 99 and fractured her pelvis, the physical therapist was impressed by the strength in her little legs. She was hospitalized twice in the past year with pneumonia and the doctor's prognosis was always grim. She surprised them both times and rebounded, heading home after two days.

My mother can still get around under her own power, with a walker, but I can see her strength starting to wane. She spends more time in her recliner, says she is tired more often than before. Sometimes she mumbles about people who are no longer living, and I wonder if she is peering into the other side.

A friend of mine who is a psychic says she has seen the spirits of my father and my grandmother visiting my mother's room.

The day after her birthday party we were talking about who attended and what we did. Because of her memory loss she has a hard time getting a picture, so I tried to describe as many details as I could, hoping one might ring a bell.

After a few minutes, she asked the date and, after telling her, I added "only 364 days till your 103rd birthday!"

She grinned, tickled by the challenge of living another year.

PART SIX: Turn Aging On Its Head

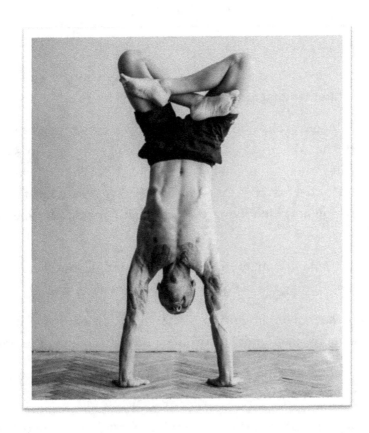

How Do I Get More Comfortable With That Face in the Mirror?

By Mary Dalton Selby

I struggle with accepting what I see. I feel younger and more vibrant than that face looking back at me!

For the last couple of years, I have been taking good care of myself. I have been eating well, working on getting quality sleep, exercising, meditating daily, and more. I was not always as diligent for the first 65 years of my life. But I've done a lot of work, researching and identifying the best health strategy for me and following it.

I have eliminated many of my vices, except alcohol. I enjoy an excellent sipping tequila or a glass of wine with dinner.

I am desperately clinging to the fact that not all of the health experts agree that moderate drinking is harmful to your brain.

I have tried looking in the mirror in the morning and telling myself that I love me just the way I am. That's not working.

My long-time partner is very accepting of my changing body, and he is even eight years younger. He has no problem with my skin sagging and hair thinning. He accepts these changes as a rite of passage. Why can't I?

What's interesting is that even though I struggle with my aging face, when I retired, I quit wearing makeup. That could be out of laziness. But I often felt the makeup was highlighting my wrinkly, saggy skin, not making it appear better.

All of my friends are getting older. I don't judge them as harshly as I do myself.

Each of my daughters has her solution for me. The oldest suggests Botox and fillers while the younger says get rid of my mirrors. She did, and she is only 34. She told me that not being exposed continuously to mirrors keeps you from spending so much time criticizing everything you see.

I still feel like I have a lot of life yet to live, places to explore and adventures to experience. It may not sound like it, but I am a happy person. I wouldn't give up my life for anything. It is just my physical manifestation that causes me such grief.

Writing has been a great source of therapy for me, an unexpected benefit. It is something I am doing just for me. It is a new project, not the voice of any of my other roles, mother, grandmother or partner, but my voice as a woman of a certain age.

The practice of writing is forcing me to organize my thoughts better and dig deeper into my feelings. I am learning a lot about myself and sharing that as I go along.

The bottom line is, I can't stop the aging process. The only thing I can control is my reaction to it. I need to quit judging this book by its cover and stop being so hard on myself. Thanks for hearing me out.

Your Attitudes About Aging Can Predict Your Future

By Brittany Denis, DPT

"One of the most interesting study findings has to do with attitudes toward aging itself. Young middle-aged people (in their forties and fifties) with positive feelings about growing older -- gaining wisdom, freedom from working, opportunities to travel and learn more -- tended to enjoy better health, and better cognitive health later in life."

Bill Gifford, health science reporter

I spend a lot of my day talking about how our attitudes impact our aging and health. Coming from a young person, I get a lot of dirty looks and people telling me I don't understand reality.

But this isn't just some delusional thinking coming from what I would like aging to be. No. Our attitudes and beliefs influencing our health as we age are backed by research.

What Research Doesn't Tell Us

The Baltimore Longitudinal Study of Aging is the longest-running study we have on aging today. It's produced a huge volume of data that's been sifted through by researchers to develop a deeper understanding of aging. Researchers have been putting subjects through a battery of tests since 1958, throughout their lifespan, to identify patterns and aging predictors.

Once researchers analyzed the data, they realized there was no single biomarker to indicate aging, which had been one of the initial intentions of the study. Nothing could be simply identified through bloodwork to tell you at what pace you would age and how much life you had left. But they did catch on to some other surprising patterns.

What It Found Instead

Participants of the study were not only subjected to physical tests but also to surveys assessing their mental health and attitudes toward aging. And one strong consistency was noted.

Middle-age adults (defined as being in their forties and fifties) who reported positive feelings about aging fared better later in life than adults who reported negative feelings about aging.

That's right. Positive thinking leading to a better quality of life as we age is evidence-backed.

It reminded me of the words of Katy Bowman who wrote in her book, *Dynamic Aging: Simple Exercises for Whole-Body Mobility*, that "exercise has powerful capabilities to improve health, but so do words."

Other studies also have found that older adults who were shown positive wording associated with aging did better on physical tests than older adults exposed to negative words associated with aging.

So, if you need evidence to change your attitudes and beliefs you can find plenty of it. And it's never too late to start to use this to your advantage.

The first step is to identify how you view aging. Make note of the thoughts that run through your mind. The next and more difficult step is to actively change your thought patterns, if you found they were mostly negative. By changing your story, you can take control of your aging today.

Looking at Old in a New Way

By Maggie Fry

A friend asked me the other day if I feel like an old woman. My initial response was, "No, of course not," but then I started thinking more about the question. What does it really mean to feel old?

There is much to consider here. There is our chronological age, which pins us in a certain finite time frame. There is our internal landscape of experiences that changes over time. There is how we interact with the world at large. There are the expectations of others and their beliefs and attitudes toward us, as well as our own internalized attitudes towards ourselves.

Clearly, we can *be* old and not *feel* old.

The word *old* itself has differing connotations. It is, in one sense, a neutral word. Saying something is old doesn't paint much of a picture in the mind. Is it vintage, antique, rare, valuable? Perhaps it is broken in, comfortable, or familiar? Or is it decrepit, used up, or decaying? Old can mean so many things.

As far as chronological age, in less than a week I will be 61. I was born at the tail end of the Baby Boom. Some of the older members of my generation screamed at Beatles concerts, made love in the mud at Woodstock, protested the Vietnam War and founded the environmental movement. These things happened fifty years ago.

I don't care that some people say, "Sixty is the new forty." That is silliness. In chronological terms, I am old.

Age gives us perspective like nothing else can. If we have paid attention — and plenty of people do not — we have an impressive body of experiences from which to draw lessons and inspiration. We see ourselves in others and the joys and problems they are facing. It brings up stories we want to share.

I think experience is the main reason that most people don't become storytellers until they are older. They haven't processed enough yet.

At this moment in time, I feel optimistic and excited about the possibilities in my life, both in terms of my writing career and my personal life, probably more so than at any other time. Looking forward to new experiences and unexplored territory is generally considered a young person's prerogative, but as I look back on my youth, I remember being afraid and confused by the future. I had no idea where I wanted to go or what I wanted to do, and I agonized over every decision. I had not yet learned that failure teaches us more than success, so we should not be afraid to try.

I feel like I have honed my life to its most important parts. For me, this had to do with time. When I turned 60, I looked at the time I could reasonably expect to have left to me — no guarantees, of course — and found some things worth pursuing and others not.

For example, I decided to return to the study of music, which I put aside in my youth. I also considered taking up belly dancing, but soon realized that if I worked really hard and practiced multiple hours every day, the best I could hope to be was mediocre, so I said goodbye to the silks and bangles. It had nothing to do with being *too old*; I simply didn't enjoy it as much as singing.

Growing older, we begin to recognize those things that bring us joy and focus on them. We release what no longer serves us, laying aside burdens that we realize we don't need to carry anymore. We feel as free as children on a hot day, happily shedding clothing on the way to a cool pond to go skinny dipping.

Sometimes we get to a point where we realize that nothing in life brings us joy, and then we have to decide to risk making some changes or stay where we are because we perceive the cost of change is too high.

Sometimes, the moment we become old is when we tell ourselves that this is it. This is all there is. There are no more adventures out there. And we settle into our space until we sink six feet down and they throw dirt on top of us.

When people say they feel old, they are often referring to living with pain. This could be physical pain, like the way older joints sometimes feel when they protest being asked to get up out of a chair and walk across the room. But I know people twenty and thirty years younger than I who suffer from chronic pain conditions, and I don't think they qualify as old.

It could be the pain of regret that haunts us, the feeling that we missed the chance to make a different choice. It could be the pain of loneliness, the feeling that the people and experiences we loved are passing from the world, and we are left behind, alone.

Obviously, we can't do anything about time. When we reach our 60s and 70s, we are definitely old, but that doesn't have to make us feel any particular way. We don't have to give up things we enjoy like dancing or hiking or going to concerts because the clock has ticked to a particular number.

Maybe feeling old also means being able to assess a situation quickly and accurately and not agonize over what to do. We've seen it before. Or perhaps we feel old when our children and younger friends are anxious about making their way in the world and we can reassure them because we've been through it ourselves.

As I think about my friend's question, *do I feel like an old woman*? I would have to say, "Yes, but it depends on how you define *old*." I am not in pain, either physically, mentally, or spiritually. I treasure the store of experiences I have collected over the years, and I continue to view my life as an adventure. I am not yet ready to stop looking toward the next horizon. That is what comes from feeling old.

What Does "Older" Feel Like?

By Nalini MacNab

I don't feel "old" until I look in the mirror. Always a surprise, the grey and the wrinkles. Greeted with a smile, these days, and a shake of those pale tresses.

My snow-capped pate, a result of closed salons and long delays for the organic color I order online, surprises me every time.

I do not feel *old*. But then, what does old feel like? My meditations are deeper now. My body still enjoys moving every day. Paying attention to my inputs —physical, emotional, and mental — is done by default. I am more aware of what works for this body and what doesn't. And everything is changing now for everyone.

The being inside feels vibrant, still.

This morning I recalled the day when, rolling carefully out of bed, still healing from head trauma, my excitement could not be contained. I'd drive the seven minutes to the stables, tack up a friend's horse, and pop him over a few fences, just for fun! Then, as I crept downstairs to the kitchen, my newly healing balance let me know that perhaps today was not that day...

I did not despair. Waking to that inspiration, those joyful thoughts, was FUN! My body was still up for it...on a day when more healing had happened.

Returning to the mountains this winter, I laughed at myself each time I arrived, slightly out of breath, at the top of the stairs. *Altitude*. We remember this! Body and I giggled in delight, knowing that our cardio-pulmonary response would adjust, that we needed to use extra sunscreen and to pay attention to hydration. *We've got this!* Fun!

Though I no longer train six days a week and prefer walking to those long runs I used to love (still would, if my knees would agree), stillness permeates my every moment...is that *old?* Or is it yet another phase in this play of becoming that we call life?

What does "older" feel like? I'm not sure I'll ever know. Wisdom is one thing. The chronological progression of our bodies, a given. But, *old?*

If every moment of life feels new, is there an opposite called old?

Today I woke, wondering. What will the day hold? What miracles will show up? How much fun will there be? Instead of *old*, I'd rather be *me*.

May it be a *great* day, for wonderers of all ages!

The Person I Used to Be Came for a Visit
And I realized a re-evaluation was in order

By Anna I. Smith

I'm 58. At this age, I'm feeling comfortable. Comfortable with who I am, where I am, what I stand for and what I can no longer accept. My life moves forward at a pleasant pace with sufficient variation to make it interesting and challenging but with enough familiarity for tranquillity to form roots.

I feel young enough and old enough at the same time. Smart enough but still curious. Kind enough but with the good sense to speak up when I have to.

Then I get a visit from a distant relative. My husband and I pick her up at the Greyhound station. From the moment she steps into our car I know her, even though we've never met. She is me. Me, almost four decades earlier. Her energy, her mannerisms, and her curiosity. Me, me, me.

She stays for four days. And during that time, I'm reminded of what I used to be like. But I also realize that the person I'm slowly turning back into still feels familiar. We still have a lot in common.

At 19, I was just like her. At that age, there was no distinction between dreams and plans. Dream it. Do it. Done. Repeat. When I was her age, the rewards almost always outweighed the risks. Falls, even those from dizzying heights, had few consequences. There was time for do-overs, for U-turns, for repeats and plan changes.

But at 19, certain issues took hold and wouldn't fade. Without the perspective that only comes with age, certain setbacks had a tendency to linger longer than they ought to. Back then there was no inner voice telling me that this, too, shall pass, telling me that whatever worries blanketed my mind would slowly dissolve. No, time doesn't heal all wounds. But time lets new experiences enter, giving existing worries some loving company.

Then I settled down. I became a mother. That had always been my ultimate dream and I loved every minute of it. Almost every minute of it. I became responsible and practical.

But in the blink of an eye, my children left our home to pursue their own dreams. They call it an empty nest for a reason. It's empty. And it's sad. It left a lot of time for wishing I could do it all over: "Please come back. I know what I'm doing now."

A period of readjustment followed. Changes can be painful. But, slowly, I let go of the parenting persona that for so long had been me. I rediscovered parts of myself I thought I had long ago left behind. And I began to stretch the boundaries I set for myself. I started small. I mean, tiny. Once in a while, we ate dinner in front of the TV. Crazy stuff like that.

Then my courage started to grow. My wilder side came out — the one that was hidden by responsibilities and ideas of being a good enough role model and not too cringe-causing a parent. I began walking around the house in my old, all-too-short, washed-out cotton nightgown. Stuff jiggled and cellulite showed. But I bent over without shame. We stayed up late, slept late, and ate when we wanted to. And we once again used our far too loud outdoor voices indoors because no one was asleep in the room down the hall.

Which is also why I still cried. No one was asleep in the room down the hall. But ever so slowly I began to dream —dreams built for two.

Together we began to plan the next stage of our lives. And I decided to try this writing thing. Dream it. Do it. Done. Repeat.

But I move forward with caution. I know what failing feels like. If I fall now, I land hard. And healing takes longer. I remind myself to tread gently.

Until the old me gets into my car telling me about her future dreams. Her dreams are her plans. Her plans are her dreams. With her, there is no difference. No hesitation.

She reminds me of what I left behind. Walking next to her I feel old. The discovery is an irritating reminder of what four decades have done to my soul.

When did my dreams become cautious, tattered rewrites adjusted to fit safety standards, budgets, and restricted timelines?

When she came here, reminding me of what I used to be like —
that's when.

The contrast between us is painful. Why did I not see it creeping
up on me?

And as the old version of me gets ready to board the Greyhound
bus for the trip back to her dorm, I hug her tight and thank her
for coming.

On the way back to our home I begin to examine my need to
become more. Could it be that I was so content because the
weights I've used to evaluate my wellbeing were far too light?
Could it be that the lines on my yardstick became smudged along
the way, giving me a faulty reading?

Once again, my house is quiet. The silence used to bother me.
Now I see it as a great opportunity to be still with my thoughts.
If I've changed, I can change once more — this time in reverse.
It's not too late to dream big. It's not too late to allow myself to
fail. Experience tells me I can still handle the falls and that the
falls are still worth it.

Why We Should Resist Any Urge to Join the Aging Tribe

The importance of social connections across generations.

By Zoe Berry

What do I mean by the "aging tribe?" The Oxford English Dictionary defines a tribe as *"a social division in traditional society consisting of families or communities linked by social, economic, religious, or blood ties, with a common culture and dialect."*

Recently it has occurred to me that, because of the many conversations that are taking place in social media and more widely in the press, we are forming tribes based on age.

A Generational Divide

There are divisions between generations because of differences in opinion on issues such as climate change and immigration and, in the United Kingdom, the referendum on whether to remain a member of the European Union.

Belonging to a group of like-minded people can be very comforting. We all like to see our views reinforced, but that also discourages us from challenging our personal views and fact-checking before we form opinions or make important decisions.

Some of the language is hostile. Young adults have been referred to as the "snowflake" generation, suggesting they are less resilient and over-sensitive to criticism, and young people have tweeted that "Baby Boomers" are stealing their future with selfish attitudes and conservative opinions. This does not encourage any kind of helpful dialogue or conversation.

There will always be differences in views between generations based on the perspective that different experiences might give us, and lifestyles change as society moves with the times. But the British Social Attitudes Survey in 2017 reported that *the factor most likely to have influenced voting decisions in the EU referendum was the level of education, not age.* The survey found that 80% of 18- to 34-year-olds with a degree voted to remain in the EU, as did 70% of those aged over 55.

As a District Nurse 40 years ago, I used to visit a lady who was 100 years old. Her first job involved travelling around central London in a horse and cart making deliveries to shops. Even 40 years ago, it was hard for me to imagine that happening around Piccadilly Circus! This lady's daughter had bought her a microwave so that she could prepare her own meals, but she never really got her head around this technology and always marveled at how quickly her "Michael-wave" would heat the food.

My point is that these differences in viewpoint are easy to understand but leave us with a simplified and somewhat dangerous state of affairs. They encourage ageist attitudes and, in many ways, divert attention from the real causes of the problems that exist in any society.

Making Connections

What we should be doing is engaging in open, non-threatening conversations with people having a range of opinions. If you demonstrate genuine interest in the reasons for dearly held opinions, you can learn a lot.

My 90-year-old mother recently moved into assisted living, much to her horror because she "doesn't like old people." This type of attitude, which, it seems, is not uncommon, can lead to self-imposed isolation.

We Need To Make And Maintain Social Connections As We Age. In the so-called "longevity hotspots," those areas with a higher than average proportion of people living over 100 years, a common characteristic is the importance attached by older people to having a sense of purpose and belonging in their community.

So, what can we do to avoid falling into the trap of reinforcing our unchallenged prejudices?

Taking Action

I plan to ensure that I continue socializing, not just on social media but face-to-face, with friends of a wide range of ages. How?

- Volunteer for an organization that attracts members from a wide age range, or join a group such as the Women's Institute;

- Take a class, either to learn something new or to take up exercise in any way I like;

- Do anything I can to keep myself open to new ideas and different points of view, perhaps by joining a book club, for example.

The truth is, we humans are dependent on each other and on our beautiful planet, so let's not draw unnecessary battle lines and allow ourselves to be diverted from the real solutions to the problems we face.

Fun with Boomer Barbie

Boomers who grew up with Barbie need an updated version.

By Roz Warren

If you're a girl and you're a Boomer, one thing is certain — you grew up playing with Barbies.

You dressed her up in stylish clothing (remember "Silken Flame?") complete with tiny matching shoes that were always falling off and getting chewed up by the dog. You sent her off on dates with Ken. You staged pajama-clad heart-to-hearts with Barbie's best pal, Midge.

Barbie play was designed to prepare you for the wonderful world of romance and dating. And that future was always wholesome and bright. (There was no Unplanned Pregnancy Barbie or High School Dropout Barbie.) Of course, the edgier kids could always improvise. I know one girl who, after seeing the movie "Gypsy," had her Barbies perform stripteases for her Kens. (Okay, so it was me.)

And I know of at least one future lesbian whose Barbie enjoyed marathon make-out sessions with Midge.

Barbie has been updated and modernized countless times since she first came on the scene in 1959 (although her shoes still fall off and the dog still chews them up.) These days Barbie doesn't just don cool outfits and go out on dates. She has a career!

Teacher Barbie! Pop Star Barbie! Airline Pilot Barbie! Brain Surgeon Barbie! Rabbi Barbie! Porn Star Barbie! (Okay, I made those last two up.)

But one thing about Barbie never changes. Her age. While the little girls who once played with her have grown and matured, Barbie hasn't aged a day. Now that we Boomers are seniors, we're playing Barbie again, this time with our grandchildren.

This gives me idea. I think we need a new kind of Barbie. A Barbie who, like us, *has* grown up.

When we get down on the floor to play with our grandkids, instead of a fresh-faced know-nothing who is just starting out, why not introduce the kids to a Barbie that reflects both our lives and their future?

Boomer Barbie! What better way to signal to our granddaughters that there's more to life than which outfit you've got on? And that while teenage dating is great, so is being a mature woman with a rich, full life?

This new line of AARP-aged Barbies could include:

Happily Married Barbie
Now that the kids are grown, Silver Fox Barbie and Slightly Balding Ken can re-focus on each other. Includes a Dream House with a paid-off mortgage, fat 401(k)s and matching Medicare cards.

Happily Divorced Barbie

After Barbie catches Ken and Midge making whoopee in the Dream House mud room, help her kick him to the curb and jump back into the dating pool. Assist Barbie in crafting her online profile, then dress her in tiny Eileen Fisher outfits and send her out on exciting dates!

Cougar Barbie

She may be in her sixties, but she loves those younger dudes. (For her date, just borrow Ken from your regular Barbie. She won't mind — he'll come back to her a much better lover.)

Never Married Barbie

Includes a tiny plastic vibrator, four cats, a library card, a multi-stamped passport evidencing lots of fun world travel and a tenured position at an Ivy League university.

Billionaire Barbie

Comes with three mansions, a private jet, a sexy investment advisor and an off-shore bank account.

Out and Proud Barbie

Includes a rainbow flag, a marriage license, and a Provincetown time-share with a signed Alison Bechdel original in the foyer.

Bestselling Author Barbie

Comes with hundreds of popular books translated into dozens of languages, an army of adoring fans, an impressive work ethic and more money in the bank than you can possibly imagine.

Every Boomer Barbie is slightly shorter and plumper than original Barbie, and comes with at least one ailment (bad knees, a bad back, cataracts, etc.) to *kvetch* about with the other Boomer Barbies. (The deluxe model has genuine hot flashes!)

And all of them talk, saying things like "Where did I put my glasses?" "Is it hot in here?" "Can you repeat that?" And "At least I have my health!"

The best Boomer Barbie of all?

Grandma Barbie

What better way to enjoy playing with your beloved granddaughter?

Grandma Barbie reads books, sings songs, plays pretend, makes cool snacks and gives great hugs. If you're lucky enough to be her granddaughter, you know there's nobody Grandma Barbie loves more than you. And shouldn't a cool grandma who loves you to bits be just as much fun for a little girl to play with as a vapid teenager who gets dressed up and goes out on dates?

Not only that, but Grandma Barbie's stylish yet sensible shoes will never fall off and get chewed up by the dog.

AUTHOR BIOGRAPHIES

If you like what you've read here, join us online at *Medium.com/crows-feet* and read more insightful stories by the authors in this collection.

Marie A. Bailey has an M.A. in Creative Writing from Florida State University. She blogs about writing, nature, cats and knitting at www.1writeway.com. She's been published in *Brevity*, by Nightingale & Sparrow, and in various publications on *Medium* as @marieannbailey. She currently lives in Florida.

Zoe Berry is a former nurse practitioner, nurse educator, and Queen's Nurse. She is now exploring how to age well and have the best later life. www.ageingisagift.co.uk

Beth Bruno has been writing about life and all its complexities since she was eight years old. She has relished her fifties and is looking forward to her sixties. She loves hanging out with her adult children and grandchildren, gardening, raising chickens and camping on uninhabited islands.

Kathleen Cardwell is now a freelance writer/editor based in Cincinnati, Ohio, following a 30+ year career in marketing and communications. Kathleen enjoys writing relevant and entertaining narratives, personal essays, and feature articles for magazines. Kathleen has recently started editing memoirs and family ancestry books. Her writing can be found on *Medium*.

Caroline Lucas de Braganza is a Wise Old Woman (WOW) who dreamed of writing when she retired. Caroline has published essays on a range of topics, from Emotional Health, Neuroscience, Self and Society to Spirit, dipping into humor when life gets too serious. Forever curious, Caroline vows to play with words for the rest of her days.

Brittany Denis, PT, DPT, RES-CPT is a physical therapist, movement coach, and educator empowering clients through the aging process with mindful movement. She inspires all adults to bring a growth mindset to aging in her movement studio as through writing and educating online.

Dennett was always a writer but lived in a bookkeeper's body before she found *Medium* and broke free — well, almost. She is working to work less and write more.

Katharine Esty, PhD is a practicing psychotherapist, widow, mother, grandmother, and an activist for aging well. She's on a mission to dispel myths about old age. She lives in a retirement community near Boston. Her recent book, *Eightysomethings: A Practical Guide to Letting Go, Aging Well, and Finding Unexpected Happiness*, can be purchased at Amazon.com. Visit https://www.katharineesty.com/newsletter-subscriptions to sign up for Katherine's twice monthly newsletter.

Maggie Fry lives on a small farm south of Erie, Pennsylvania, where she spends her time gardening, cooking, spinning, and writing. She also loves to travel.

J. F. Gross is a graduate of The University of Missouri School of Journalism and worked for more than 30 years for newspapers in Colorado. She is now retired in Flagstaff, Arizona.

Greg Hopkins lives in Italy with his wife Chrissy and their dog Tilda. Greg is endlessly fascinated by the paradox of perfection, wholeness and healing in the midst of chaos.

Paul Hossfield is a retired engineer living in the diminutive yet great state of Rhode Island. Until March of 2020 he was quite active. Now he stays home, makes masks, writes under the pseudonym Quasimodo on *Medium*, finds useful things to do when possible, and gets about chiefly by bicycle.

Julia E. Hubbel, when not out traveling the backwoods of the world, may be found cleaning the blackberries out of her yard in Oregon. Or writing. She's pretty good at writing, very good at riding horses, and really, really good at making fun of aging.

Ann Litts is a 60-year-old mother and grandmother who loves J.R.R. Tolkien, black coffee, good tequila, and losing at Candy Land. A nurse for over 25 years, she looks forward to retirement with much anticipation and joie-de-vivre. Nature is her church. She doesn't write, she listens and then shares the message The Universe dictates to whomever needs to hear it.

Nalini McNab is an internationally recognized author, blogger, wisdom teacher and transformational seer. She is the author of several books, including *Walk A New Way* and *The Samurai Scotties* trilogy. She is not affiliated with any group, organization or religion. Find her work at www.goddessportalsupport.com and on *Medium.com/@chaliceofwisdom*.

Shea McNaughton is a city girl living in the country doing country stuff and loving every bit of it. She says she needs two lifetimes to do all she wants to do. Blogger, photographer, world traveler, reader, dancer, and now biker chick.

Donna McNicol retired as an IT professional and started writing fiction. Her preferred genre is small town mysteries with a dash of romance, but she has also tackled children's stories, fantasy and small-town romance. Her short stories have been included in several anthologies. She lives in rural Tennessee with her husband and two Goldendoodles. Please visit Donna at https://campsite.bio/dbmcnicol to follow her.

Michelle Monet is a musician, author, poet, and seeker. She is currently writing a showbiz memoir and Broadway style Musical. Contact her at michelle@michellemonet.com

Diane Overcash is a fine art painter, fiddler, actor and arranger of words. She is also a butter snob.

Nancy Peckenham is the editor of *Crow's Feet*, which she started after a career in journalism. She writes about life as we age, travel adventures, history and matters of the human spirit.

Lili Rodriguez is a native New Yorker who has lived on a farm in Hawaii with two life partners and a bunch of critters (including four very loud parrots) since 1999. Over 60 herself, Lili is a cultural anthropologist, consumer researcher, entrepreneur and wannabe writer. She is fascinated by life's surprising complexity and obsessed with understanding the "why" behind the "what."

Anne Saddler lives in a lively Cornish port in the UK. After a career writing primarily non-fiction, Anne has returned to her first love, poetry and fiction writing. Her book *North Of The Heart,* a selection of poetry and prose, is available from Amazon books world-wide (paperback and Kindle).

Mary Dalton Selby, who is retired and living in the Midwest, transitioned from a career in the digital world to playing on the floor with her grandkids. Retirement has also given her the opportunity to explore new interests, like writing.

Anna I. Smith writes about relationships and situations that make her laugh, cry or both. When not writing she loves to bake, watch movies and analyze the state of the world and everything in it. She lives in Southern California with her husband, her pets, and other wild and crazy animals.

Mark Starlin is a musician and writer who began his writing adventure at the age of 57. He recently turned 60. His writing spans a wide variety of topics and genres, including fiction, humor, poetry, and essays. He has published one novel, a collection of fiction, and a collection of humor.

Warren Turner is a semi-retired progressive clergyperson who writes personal essays about life at 80. Warren is a Minnesota Twins fan and supporter of all LGBTQ+ issues. He/Him.

Roz Warren, Medium Sherpa and writing coach, writes for everyone from the *New York Times* to the *Funny Times*. She is the author of several books, including *Our Bodies, Our Shelves: A Collection Of Library Humor* (Humour Outcast Press, 2015).

Lisa Wathen lives in southeast Virginia with her family and cat and teaches high school English and journalism. She has published a children's book and short YA fiction and is currently working on several MG and YA novels, including an anthology of ghost stories. Her short adult fiction and nonfiction work is available on *Medium*.

Ingrid L. Williams is an unrepentant writer specializing in storytelling with purpose and impact. With over 20 years of experience ranging from international journalism and brand-building to marketing and storytelling, she has written or contributed to a number of articles, books, scripts, commercials, presentations, videos, speeches, mixed reality entertainment and other formats.

ACKNOWLEDGMENTS

I want to thank my husband, Mark, who has encouraged me to write about life as we age since we first got to know the residents of a senior living residence. His support of my work has been unflinching, and his insights have inspired my thinking about age. My mother, Catherine, also provided great inspiration, with her unending enthusiasm for life.

This book would not exist with the scores of writers who are willing to share their own personal stories on *Medium*, stories that tell of the joys of aging as well as the difficulties they face because of ageism. I want to thank each and every one of them.

Finally, I would like to thank Marne Platt, who provided the vital editing support to bring this collection over the finish line.

CPSIA information can be obtained
at www.ICGtesting.com
Printed in the USA
LVHW020239301120
673004LV00038B/1092